Jin Shin *for* Cats *and* Dogs

"An easy-to-digest manual for cat and dog owners, tackling small as well as more complex topics, whether they are based on health-related or psychological issues. The images and step-by-step instructions allow also those new to this practice to optimally use the correct hand positions to help their pet."

– MELANIE KESSLER, alternative practitioner and Reiki healer for
animals and animal psychologist and communicator

"I highly recommend Tina Stümpfig's *Jin Shin for Cats and Dogs*. It is fun to read and the handholds are easy to use. As with humans, you can also activate the self-healing properties of dogs and cats. From physical to psychological problems all is well explained, and the additional use of images makes it easy to understand and thereby suitable for beginners as well as those more advanced."

– KIRSTEN MOHR, animal Jin Shin practitioner

"Every pet owner dreams of an easy, gentle method without side effects that enables them to help their sick dog or ailing cat themselves. The healing flow of Jin Shin Jyutsu makes this possible—simply by touching specific points and areas on the body. Holding certain 'safety energy locks' activates energy flows, releases blockages, and thus paves the path to maintaining or restoring health. You can learn how easy and straightforward this is in Tina Stümpfig's *Jin Shin for Cats and Dogs*. Her book does not stop at physical ailments only: she also gives useful therapeutic advice on behavioral disorders and psychic problems. An absolute must for every dog- and cat-loving person who wants to help their pet themselves or effectively accompany a veterinarian therapy."

– MONIKA FALCK, animal communicator and
family constellator with animals

Jin Shin *for* CATS *and* DOGS

Healing Touch for Your Animal Companions

TINA STÜMPFIG

 FINDHORN PRESS

Findhorn Press
One Park Street
Rochester, Vermont 05767
www.findhornpress.com

Findhorn Press is a division of Inner Traditions International

Disclaimer
The information in this book is given in good faith and is neither intended to diagnose
any physical or mental condition nor to serve as a substitute for informed medical
advice or care. Please contact your health professional for medical advice and treatment.
Neither author nor publisher can be held liable by any person for any loss or damage
whatsoever which may arise from the use of this book or any of the information therein.

Cataloging-in-Publication Data for this title is available from the Library of Congress

ISBN 978-1-64411-459-9 (print)
ISBN 978-1-64411-460-5 (ebook)

Printed and bound in the United States by Versa Press, Inc.

10 9 8 7 6 5 4 3 2 1

Edited by Jacqui Lewis
Text design and layout by Damian Keenan
This book was typeset in Calluna, Calluna Sans,
with Editor Condensed used as a display typeface.

To send correspondence to the author of this book, mail a first-class letter to the
author c/o Inner Traditions • Bear & Company, One Park Street, Rochester,
VT05767, USA, and we will forward the communication, or contact the author
directly at **www.tinastuempfig.de**.

Contents

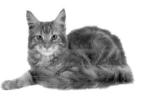

JIN SHIN HEALING TOUCH FOR CATS

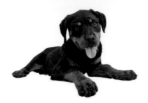

JIN SHIN HEALING TOUCH FOR DOGS

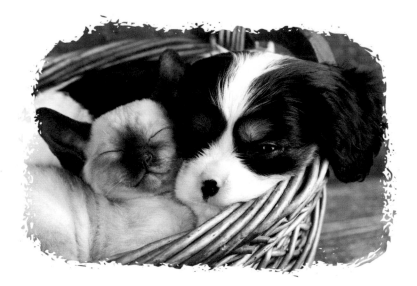

Preface

Jin Shin Jyutsu is a form of intuitive healing knowledge that all we humans carry inside us from birth and often unconsciously use time and again.

When we put our heads in our hands while thinking, for example, we activate certain parts of our brain and thereby help ourselves to remember things. At school, children often sit on their hands, which helps them to focus, to listen more carefully and to remember what they have learned. When we cross our arms, we touch a point in the crook of the elbow, which helps to align us with our own authority and power. We also intuitively place our hands on painful areas, on ourselves or on an animal, as a means of reassurance. Everyone knows Jin Shin Jyutsu—we just need to remember it again.

Jin Shin Jyutsu is a gentle healing art to harmonize life energy, which can be applied to humans as well as animals. By placing our hands on certain points on the body, life energy is brought back into flow, self-healing potentials are stimulated, and complaints and symptoms are alleviated or completely eliminated. Holding Jin Shin points is a wonderful and easy way to regain mental and physical balance.

You can use Jin Shin Jyutsu to help your cat or dog, if they are undergoing veterinary treatment or are about to have an operation. Jin Shin Jyutsu has a strengthening effect after surgical interventions, supports the healing process and makes it easier to tolerate anesthetics.

By holding certain points on the body, you help to "jump-start" life energy so that it can flow harmoniously, evenly and powerfully again. Health and well-being rely on this harmonious flow of life energy.

Even if your cat or dog has no symptoms or other issues, you can use the flows as a preventative measure. You can strengthen the health and resilience of your pet with just a few minutes of treatment.

This book gives you the opportunity to use the wonderful method of Jin Shin Jyutsu—which is essentially much more than a method—effortlessly and without prior knowledge. Enjoy the art of Jin Shin Jyutsu with your pets!

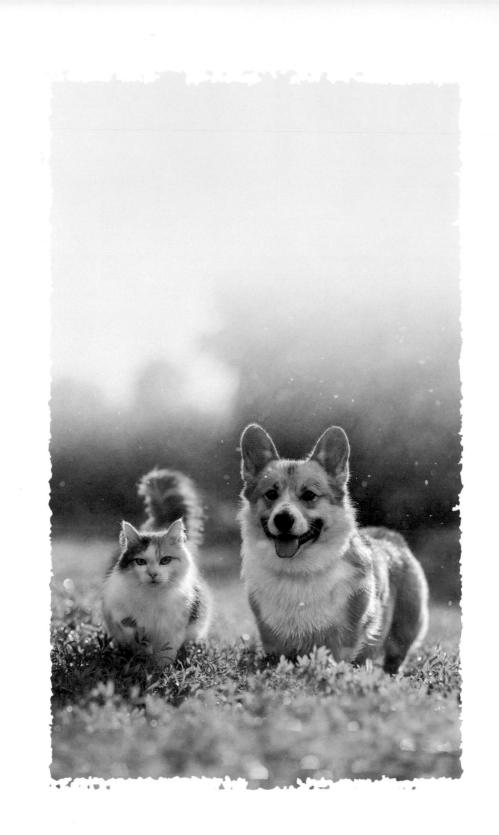

Introduction to Jin Shin Healing

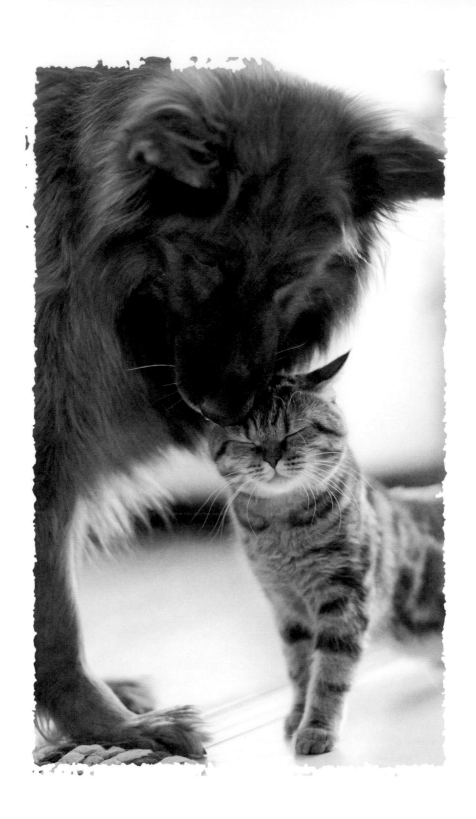

What Is Jin Shin Jyutsu?

Jin Shin Jyutsu is an ancient art for harmonizing life energy in the body. When life energy flows harmoniously, humans and animals are healthy. When blockages arise in the energy pathways, these manifest in the form of discomfort and initial symptoms. If energy remains out of balance, these symptoms can become entrenched, chronic, and new ones may appear.

The ancient knowledge of Jin Shin healing touch was embodied, applied and orally transmitted in different cultures in earlier times, until it was finally forgotten in the course of time. In the Far East, however, this valuable knowledge was not completely lost, and hence it was a Japanese man, Jiro Murai, who brought this valuable art back to life at the beginning of the twentieth century. He named it "Jin Shin Jyutsu" and passed it on to his pupils Kato Sensei and Mary Burmeister.

The term "Jin Shin Jyutsu" consists of three Japanese words:
- *Jin: knowing, compassionate person*
- *Shin: creator*
- *Jyutsu: art*

and means *"The Art of the Creator through the Knowing, Compassionate Person."*

In colloquial terms, Jin Shin Jyutsu is described as "harmonizing energy flows," since the holding of certain energy points on the body stimulates life energy to "flow" freely again, and this can be felt with a little practice. These energy points, where energy is present in a highly concentrated form, are called "safety energy locks." There are a total of 26 of these points in the body. When these points are held, blockages can be easily released. These safety energy locks are located within the energy pathways that bring life into the body. If blockages arise in these pathways, the flow of energy in the respective area is interrupted and ultimately the entire energy flow pattern is disrupted. Then disharmony and illness arise.

■ *By placing your hands on certain safety energy locks, you can support your cat or dog to regain harmony mentally, physically and psychologically, as blockages dissolve and symptoms disappear.*

The Application of Jin Shin Jyutsu

Originally, Jin Shin Jyutsu was rediscovered for humans. However, energetic laws apply equally to animals and so we can use it for cats and dogs as well. Often animals actually react more quickly to being treated than humans, as they have a different energy vibration; and, perhaps also because they do not get in their own way with mental blocks.

While for humans the following rules apply: treatment for an adult—approximately one hour, for a child—approximately 20–30 minutes, for animals it is 10–15 minutes—often even less. Pets tend to show you clearly when treatments are enough by simply moving away from you.

In general, to apply Jin Shin Jyutsu you hold two points on the body at the same time, usually two safety energy locks. Place your fingers or the palm of your hand on the indicated points until life energy begins to flow freely again. You can feel this, as a kind of tingling sensation, an inner flow or a steady pulsation. Everyone may perceive this a little differently. All you need to do is hold these points. You do not give of your own energy. Instead your hands serve as jumper cables, so to speak, so that "energy batteries" can be recharged and life energy can flow freely and powerfully again.

Hold the indicated points with your fingers, fingertips or palms until you feel a steady flow or pulsation. In the beginning, when you are new to this experience, this pulsation or flow is often not clearly noticeable. It can take a while to attune to the subtle energies and to perceive them clearly. In the meantime, just keep to the following rule: hold each point or combined points for 1–3 minutes, and then move on to the next. If you are only harmonizing one point, you can hold it for 10–15 minutes.

With a longer flow like the main central flow, which consists of seven steps, it is sufficient if you maintain each hold for two minutes so that your pet is treated for about 15 minutes at a time. However, you can also keep to shorter sequences and give treatments more often during the day. Your pets will usually show you when it is enough by turning away from you, becoming restless, or just walking away. Sometimes this is the case after less than one minute. That is perfectly fine. Simply give them another treatment later.

Helpful Hints

Quick Guide to Holding Points

- Make sure that the atmosphere is as calm and undisturbed as possible.
- Feed your cat or dog beforehand so that they are not hungry and their physical needs do not disturb the peace.
- Decide which points or flows to use.
- To start off, hold the initial centering points (p. 17).
- Then place your hands or fingers on the chosen energy points.
- Hold the points until you feel a calm, even flow or pulsation (2–3 minutes per hold).
- Depending on the issue at hand, you can give 2–3 treatments—or more—per day. Your pets will show you what is best for them.
- There are different safety energy locks or flows for most issues. Try them out, see what feels good. If your pet does not like a certain hold, try another.
- You cannot go wrong!

Relax

Jin Shin Jyutsu is effortless. Let go of all strain and effort. It can be easy! Just pay attention to what is good for you and your pet. Instead of paying attention to symptoms and to eliminating them, focus on harmony and the life energy that is always there. Feel the pulse that brings life into the body and maintains a perfect energy cycle. Through your treatments you strengthen this pulse. And you harmonize the energy flows that create, nourish and renew the body. Let your intuition guide you to find your own way. Once again: you cannot go wrong! Even if you accidentally hold a "wrong" point, there are no negative consequences. It may just take a little longer for your treatment to have an impact. The harmonizing of energy flows is always linked to the intelligence of the body, and the body ultimately uses the harmonized energy exactly as is needed.

Keep Going

In cases of more severe or chronic illnesses, it is particularly important to harmonize energy points regularly. You can simply give treatments for a few minutes at a time throughout the day, thus offering regular impulses to the body. Alternatively, you can hold points for a little longer once a day. Let your pet guide you, depending on what it is comfortable with. And, remember: healthy cats and dogs like to be treated too! Regular treatments allow your pet to drop into a deep state of relaxation, in which extensive regeneration and healing can take place.

Be Patient

If initially you notice no change with respect to a certain issue that you are treating, do not let yourself be disturbed. The body's system usually first regulates what the living organism needs most. Perhaps your pet has become calmer and more relaxed overall, or perhaps another symptom has suddenly disappeared—Jin Shin Jyutsu always works, even if we are not aware of it ourselves.

However, this does not imply that it is meant to replace a doctor. Always get a check-up from a vet if your cat or dog is weak, sick or injured. You can then always offer additional support by harmonizing energy points.

Have confidence, relax, avoid putting yourself under pressure and enjoy your time with your pet. Be curious about the effect, which can sometimes occur very quickly—and at other times happens in ways that we did not expect. Every treatment brings more harmony, strengthens the immune system and stimulates self-healing capacities.

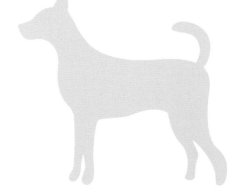

The 26 Safety Energy Locks

The energy locks, also known as safety energy locks (short: SEL), are, as mentioned already, certain points on the body where energy is present in a highly concentrated form. They are places of high conductivity that, when touched, transmit a given stimulus to the entire energy flow pattern or energy pathways.

The 26 safety energy locks are arranged symmetrically on each side of the body. Below are the images of the **SEL-placements** in cats and dogs.

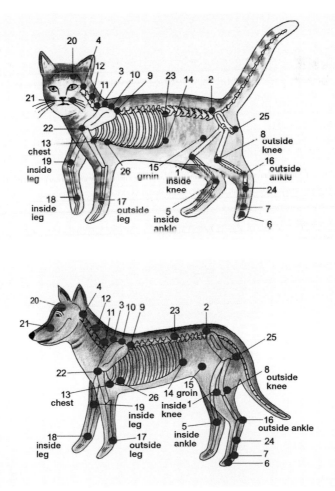

The diameter of each SEL corresponds more or less to the size of a paw—and in humans, to that of a hand. This means you do not need to worry about actually locating a point, as it is big enough. Nevertheless, if you do not manage to locate a point precisely at first, it is not a big deal. You will find that you will increasingly internalize the location of the **SELs** over time and eventually you will accurately locate them of your own accord.

Since you can not go wrong with harmonizing energy points, and with this being more of an art than a technique (you are the artist!), just experiment, give it a go, see what feels good, and what relaxes your cat or dog. There are several ways to treat any one symptom or issue. Be creative, let your gut instinct guide you. Trust yourself and your pet—intuitively, they often know very well what they need in any given moment.

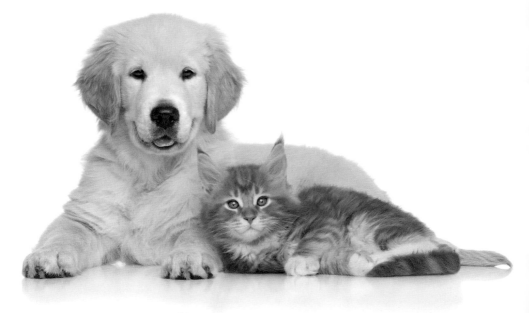

General Harmonizers

The following hold is very suitable for starting a treatment:

Place one hand on **SEL 13**, the other hand on **SEL 10**.

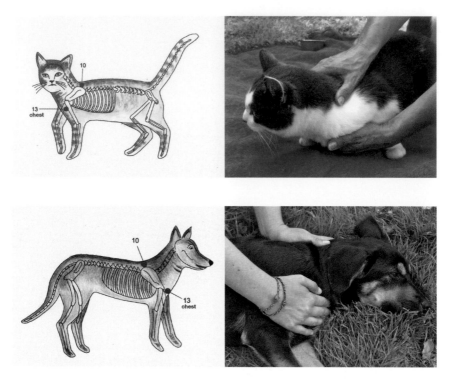

This is a good hold to say hello, to attune and to begin to relax. It brings the exhale and inhale into balance, facilitates a state of rest and fosters engagement with the treatment.

This is an important hold for

- all breathing issues,
- allergies,
- coughs,
- chest colds (bronchitis),
- pregnancy,
- neglected and abused pets,
- and very shy animals.

GETTING THE ENERGY FLOWING

This simple hold is also good for initiating a treatment. It gets energy flowing and at the same time has a deeply calming effect. It is also a helpful hold for very restless cats or dogs that generally do not like to be touched. *Likewise, it is a good first aid hold for all injuries, accidents, shock and overheating.*

For the left side of the body:

Place the *left hand* on the left **SEL 4** (directly under the base of the skull) and the *right hand* on the left **SEL 13** (on the left side of the chest, approximately at the height of the third rib).

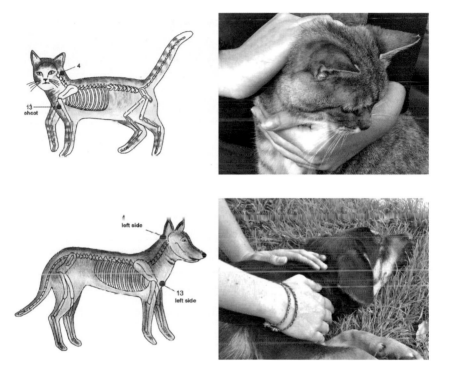

And reverse this for the right side of the body:

Right hand on the right **SEL 4** and *left hand* on the right **SEL 13**. This hold

- harmonizes emotions,
- dispels general fatigue,
- helps with everything related to the head,
- strengthens the eyes,
- supports the legs on the corresponding side of the body,
- helps the hips and is very helpful for end of life support (see pp. 136 & 220).

THE PAW FLOW

The paw flow corresponds to the finger–toe flow for humans. For this flow, always hold a finger with the opposite toe on the other side of the body. In other words, the thumb of the *right hand* and the *left small toe*, the *right index finger* and the *second smallest left toe*, etc.

For the paw flow for cats and dogs hold the entire paw: one front paw and the rear paw on the other side of the body, i.e., the right front paw with the left rear paw and the left front paw with the right rear paw. This is a very simple, yet extremely effective flow that can be used anywhere and anytime.

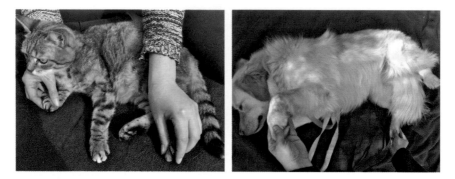

The paw flow regenerates and renews the entire body, helps with broken bones and sprains, strengthens the spine and helps with all back issues. *It is an important flow in the event of a stroke and serves as a first aid hold for injuries.*

THE MAIN CENTRAL FLOW

The main central flow connects humans and animals directly with the universal source of life, with divine energy, with the source that brings life into the body. It is also called "miracle healer" or "main central vertical flow" and it supplies humans and animals with universal life energy. It flows uninterruptedly down the front of our body, down the belly of animals, and up again on the back or top of the body respectively; in other words, it flows exactly down the center line of the body, hence the name "central flow."

Jiro Murai also called this flow the "great breath of life." As a direct connection to universal energy, it is, so to speak, our main source of energy supply, the connection between spirit and matter. Life is only possible through this flow. It provides the energy for all processes in the body.

By holding certain energy points we can help the central flow circulate freely and powerfully. Do not let the length of this flow put you off. You will notice right from the start how logical and simple the holds of this flow are.

As it is the most powerful flow there is, it is definitely worth engaging with time and again. Hold the points of this flow by sitting on the left side of your pet. It is not as complicated as it looks.

STEP 1: Place your *left hand* between the two **SELs 13** in the middle of the chest. Leave it there until the end of the flow. Place your *right hand* in the middle of both **SELs 25**, i.e., at the lower end of the spine.

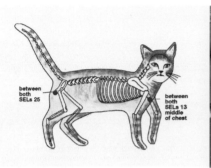

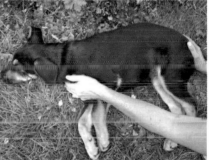

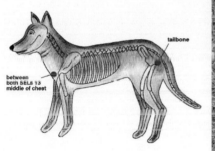

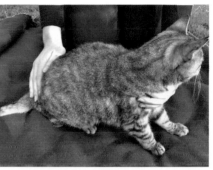

STEP 2: Place your *right hand* in the middle of both **SELs 2** on the upper edge of the pelvis.

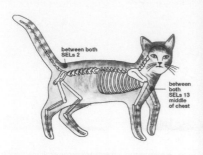

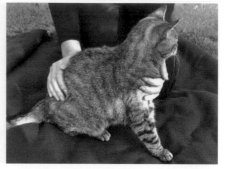

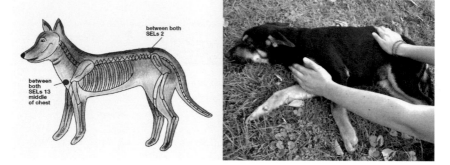

STEP 3: Place your *right hand* in the middle of both **SELs 23**, i.e., on the back at the level of the last costal arch.

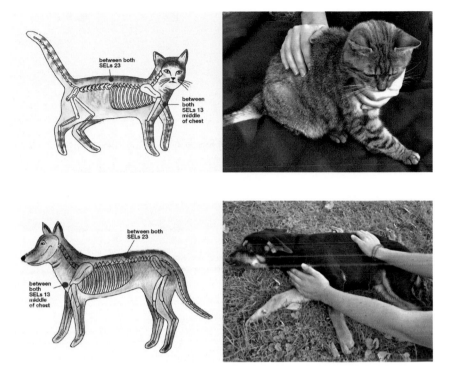

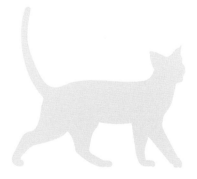

STEP 4: Place your *right hand* in the middle of both **SELs 9**, **10** and **3**, between the shoulder blades.

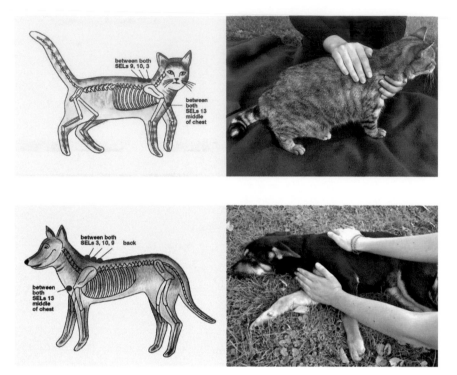

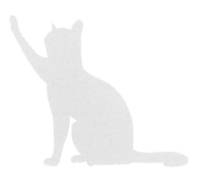

STEP 5: Place your *right hand* in the middle of both **SELs 11** at the lower end of the cervical vertebrae.

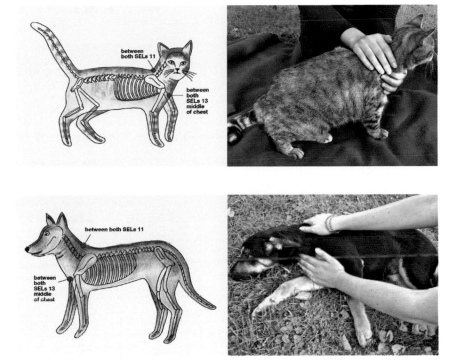

STEP 6: Place your *right hand* in the middle of both **SELs 12**, i.e., in the middle of the neck.

With bigger dogs you can in a second step place your *right hand* in the middle of both **SELs 4**, directly under the base of the skull.

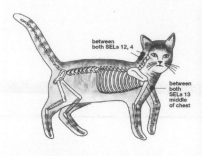
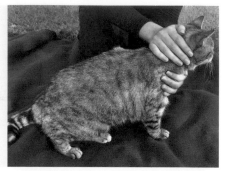

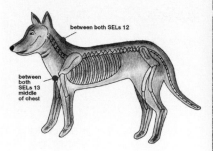
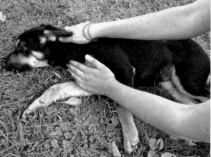

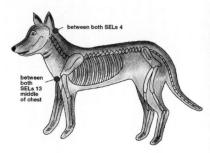
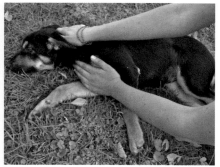

STEP 7: Place your *right hand* in the middle of both **SELs 20**, in the middle of the forehead.

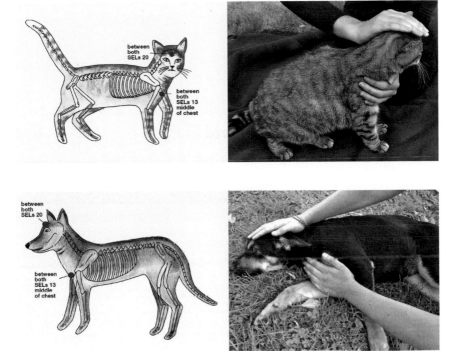

The main central flow is very powerful—it brings the whole living being into harmony and balance by furthering complete regeneration.

The Main Central Flow

- relaxes body, psyche and nerves,
- brings new energy to body, mind and soul,
- supports the immune system,
- harmonizes the hormonal system,
- stimulates the metabolism, activates self-healing capacities,
- can heal deep trauma,
- can dissolve fears and depression,
- strengthens the spine,
- has a positive effect on the nervous system, the heart and the circulatory system and it promotes harmonization from head to toe.

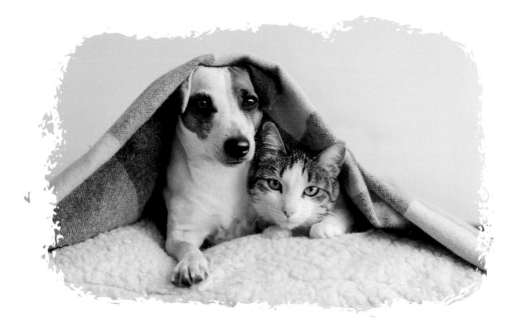

THE SUPERVISOR FLOWS

The supervisor flows also harmonize the whole being. They are two energy pathways that run symmetrically along the left and right sides of the body.

The name comes from their task, which is to look after and support both sides of the body—and, at the same time, to support all **SELs** located on these pathways. The supervisor flows, just like the main central flow, have a very deep and comprehensive effect.

You can use the holds described below for general harmonization and also when you are not really sure what to harmonize. They help every time and with everything.

Application on the left side of the body:

STEP 1: Place one hand on the left **SEL 11** (lower end of the cervical spine) and the other hand on the left **SEL 25** (under the hindquarters).

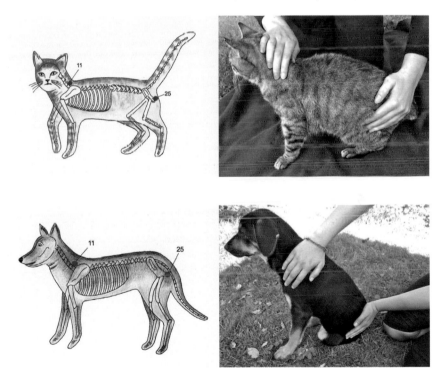

STEP 2: Keep one hand on the left **SEL 11**, and place the other hand on the left **SEL 15** (in the groin).

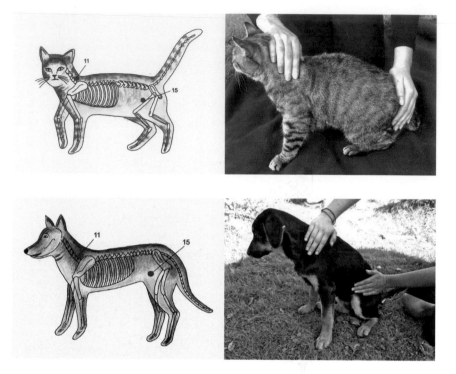

For the right side of the body reverse the hold:

STEP 1: Place one hand on the right **SEL 11** and the other hand on the right **SEL 25**.

STEP 2: Keep one hand on the right **SEL 11** and place the other hand on the right **SEL 15**.

The Supervisor Flows

- can always be applied,
- strengthen the entire energy system and harmonize the whole being,
- harmonize breathing,
- support digestion,
- strengthen the spine,
- promote the healing of broken bones,
- help to reduce stress,
- support and harmonize all **SELs**,
- and are very helpful in all critical situations.

Three Further Important Flows

In Jin Shin Jyutsu there are three other important energy pathways that also have a very powerful and profound effect, namely these organ flows: the spleen flow, the stomach flow and the bladder flow.

When I speak of organ flows, I am referring not only to the organ itself, but also to the energy quality that is connected to this organ, i.e., the associated physical and psychological counterparts that go beyond the organ.

You can treat the side of the body that is particularly in need, where the symptom appears or is more severe. Alternatively, you can treat both sides of the body one after the other. Even if you only treat one side of the body, this impacts the other side too.

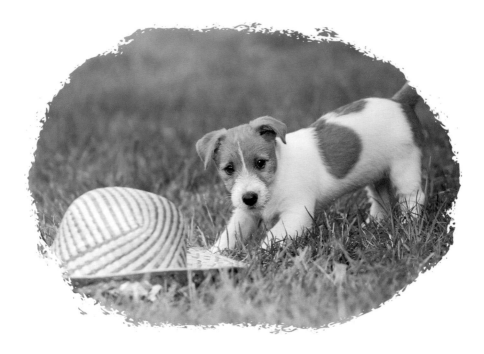

THE SPLEEN FLOW

The spleen is also known as the "place of laughter" and the spleen flow as our "personal sunbed." The spleen flow is the most important flow for the immune system. It renews the entire body and supplies all organs with energy. It strengthens the core and helps us trust life. It also opens the solar plexus and nourishes all other flows.

The Spleen Flow
- is an important flow for pets that have been through a lot of suffering,
- dissolves deep fears and evokes profound trust in life,
- heals trauma,
- relieves stress and nervousness,
- reduces hypersensitivity,
- balances emotions,
- relieves deep fears,
- furthers profound trust,
- strengthens the immune system,
- helps with hypersensitivity and nervousness,
- supports the skin,
- helps with allergies,
- supports blood formation,
- strengthens the connective tissue,
- has a supportive effect in cases of tumors,
- and assists the spleen.

Application on the left side of the body:
STEP 1: Place your *right hand* on the left **SEL 5** (on the inside of the leg at the ankle) and the *left hand* on the coccyx (lower end of the spine).

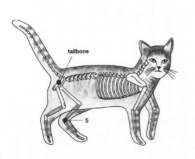

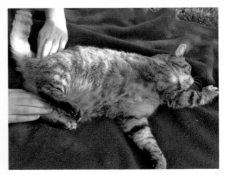

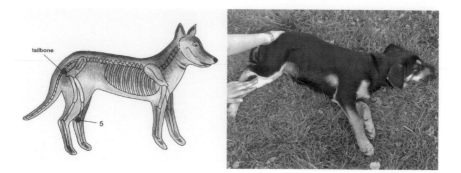

Left hand remains on the coccyx, the *right hand* moves to the right **SEL 14** (below the last costal arch).

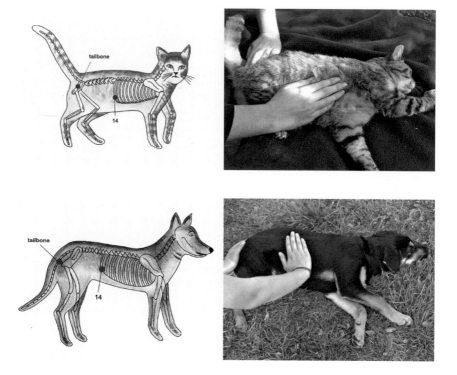

STEP 3: The *right hand* remains on the right **SEL 14**, the *left hand* moves to the left **SEL 13** (on the left side of the chest just below the third rib).

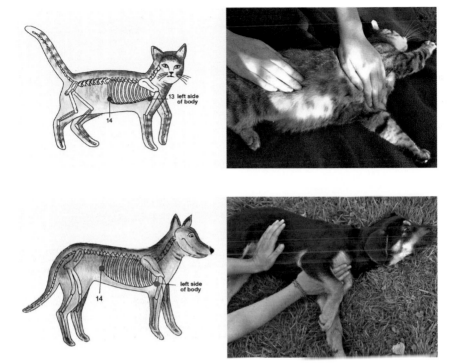

STEP 4: The *right hand* remains on the right **SEL 14**, while the *left hand* moves to the right **SEL 22** (under the right collarbone).

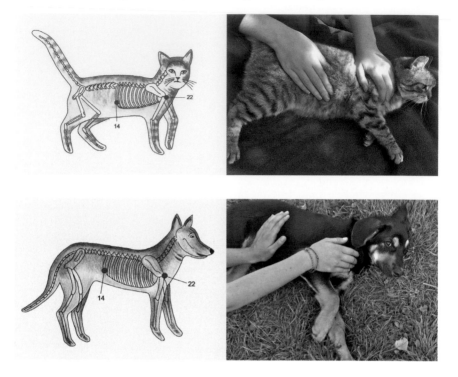

For the right side of the body, reverse the holds:

STEP 1: Place the *left hand* on the right **SEL 5** and the *right hand* on the tailbone (base of the tail).

STEP 2: The *right hand* remains on the tailbone, and the *left hand* moves to the left **SEL 14**.

STEP 3: The *left hand* remains on the left **SEL 14** while the *right hand* moves to the right **SEL 13**.

STEP 4: The *left hand* remains on the left **SEL 14**, and the *right hand* moves to the left **SEL 22**.

Quickie for the spleen flow:

First step of the spleen flow (p. 35).

The stomach flow runs along the underside of the body from the head to the hind paws. It keeps the center open so that energy can flow freely down the body and up again. The stomach flow clears and harmonizes from head to toe. Do not let the length of the flow put you off!

The Stomach Flow

- helps with digestive issues,
- and with abdominal pain and colic,
- harmonizes diarrhea (left flow) and constipation (right flow),
- relieves bloating,
- brings weight and appetite into balance,
- helps with everything that has to do with the skin and coat,
- and with allergies,
- is important for the head area (jaws, lips, teeth, gums, nose, sinuses, ears),
- reduces the excessive flow of saliva,
- helps with worries and fears,
- is supportive when pets demand an extreme amount of attention,
- helps with nervousness and "tics,"
- promotes hormonal balance,
- regulates muscle tone,
- has a harmonizing effect on diabetes,
- supports the kidneys,
- and helps to digest everything—whether physical or emotional.

Application on the left side of the body:

STEP 1: Place your *left hand* on the left **SEL 21** (on the lower edge of the zygomatic bone just above the nose) or alternatively, if your pet does not like being touched on the face, on the left **SEL 12** (on the side of the neck in the middle of the cervical spine). This hand remains there for the entire flow. The *right hand* moves to the left **SEL 22** (under the left collarbone). In the photos, **SEL 12** is being treated.

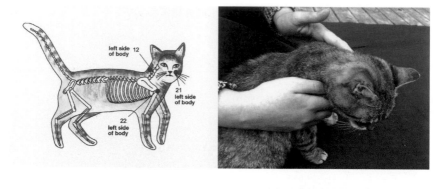

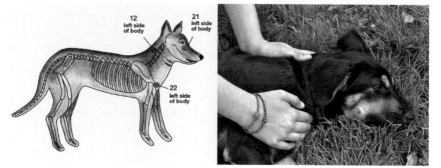

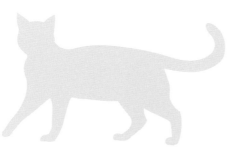

STEP 2: The *right hand* moves to the right **SEL 14** (laterally below the last costal arch on the right side).

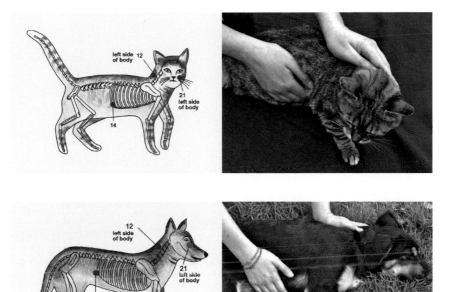

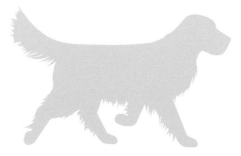

STEP 3: Now the *right hand* moves to the right **SEL 23** (between the last costal arch and the spine).

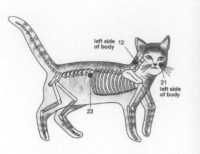
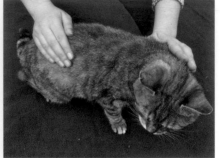

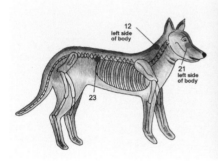
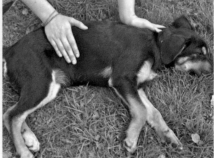

STEP 4: Place your *right hand* on the left **SEL 14** (laterally below the last costal arch).

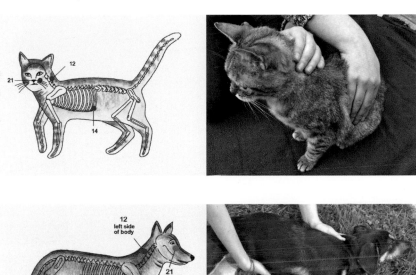

STEP 5: Place your *right hand* on the right high **SEL 1** (inside of the hind leg a little above the knee joint).

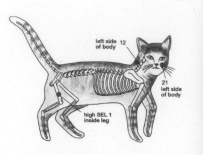

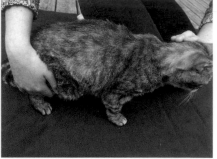

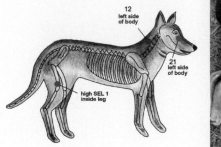

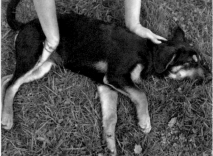

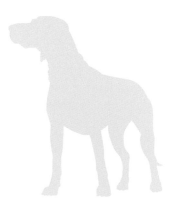

STEP 6: Place your *right hand* on the right low **SEL 8** (outside of the back leg a little below the knee joint).

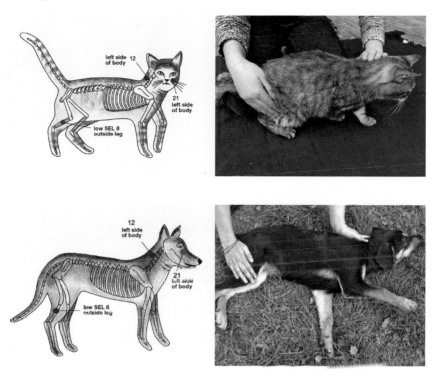

STEP 7: Now hold the right hind paw with your *right hand*.

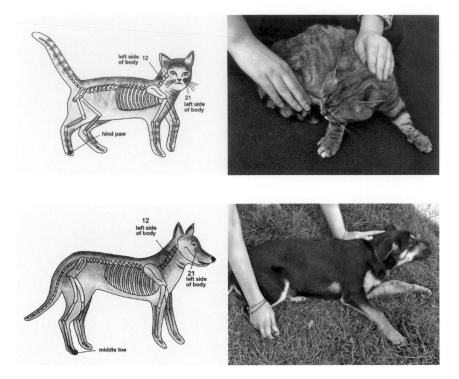

For the right side of the body, reverse the holds:

STEP 1: Place your *right hand* on the right **SEL 21**, or alternatively on the right **SEL 12**, where it remains for the entire flow. The *left hand* moves to the right **SEL 22**.

STEP 2: The *left hand* moves to the left **SEL 14**.

STEP 3: Now the *left hand* moves to the left **SEL 23**.

STEP 4: Place your *left hand* on the right **SEL 14**.

STEP 5: Place your *left hand* on the left high **SEL 1**.

STEP 6: Place your *left hand* on the left deep **SEL 8**.

STEP 7: Hold the left hind paw with your *left hand*.

Quickie for the Stomach Flow:

Place one hand on **SEL 22** and the other hand on **SEL 14**.

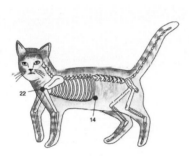

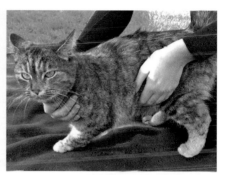

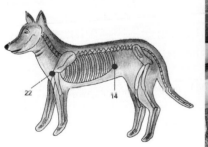

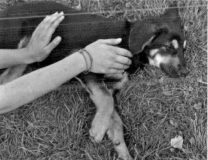

The bladder flow is a very simple flow. All holds are on the same side of the body and easy to reach.

The Bladder Flow

- has a balancing and harmonizing effect,
- is very helpful for pets that come from an animal shelter,
- gives deep inner security and serenity,
- brings peace and balance,
- harmonizes envy and jealousy,
- supports the bladder, so it can be used for all bladder issues,
- helps the back,
- harmonizes muscles (sore, weak, tense muscles and when building up muscles),
- supports weak heart muscles,
- helps with edema,
- reduces pain in the body,
- helps knees and calves,
- supports detoxification and elimination,
- harmonizes diarrhea and constipation,
- helps with rheumatic diseases,
- is helpful before and after castration,
- harmonizes fears and strengthens trust.

Application on the left side of the body:

STEP 1: Place your *left hand* on the left **SEL 12** (next to the spine in the middle of the neck). The *left hand* remains there during the entire flow. Place your *right hand* on the tailbone (lower end of the spine).

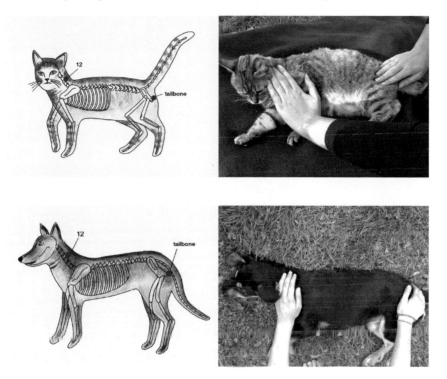

STEP 2: Place your *right hand* on the left **SEL 8** (outside of the hind leg at the knee joint).

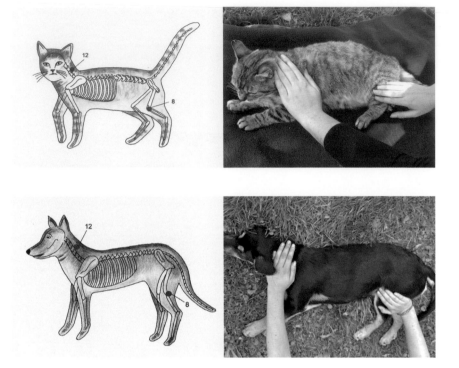

STEP 3: Place your *right hand* on the left **SEL 16** (on the outside of the ankle).

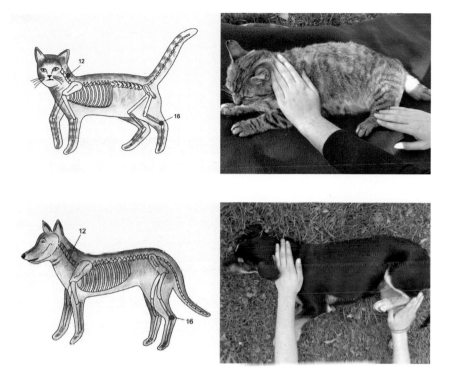

STEP 4: Hold the left hind paw with your *right hand*.

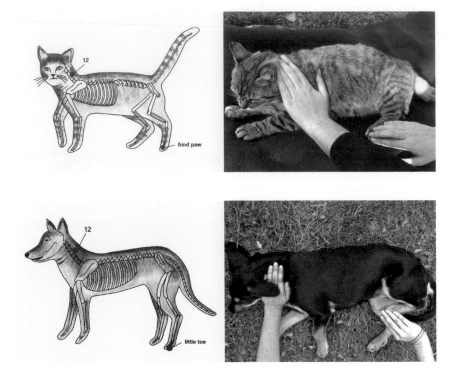

And vice versa for the right side of the body:

STEP 1: Place your *right hand* on the right **SEL 12**. It remains there during the entire flow. Put your *left hand* on the tailbone.

STEP 2: Place your *left hand* on the right **SEL 8**.

STEP 3: Place your *left hand* on the right **SEL 16**.

STEP 4: Hold the right back paw with your *left hand*.

Quickie for the bladder flow:

Place one hand on **SEL 12** and the other hand on **SEL 23**.

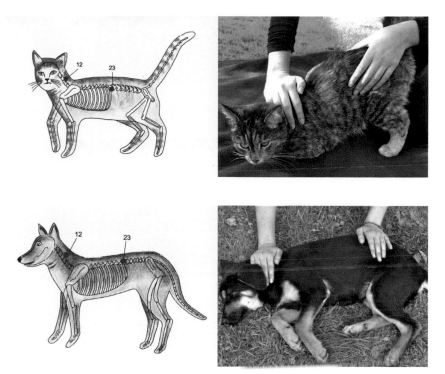

Or place one hand on **SEL 23** and the other hand on **SEL 25**.

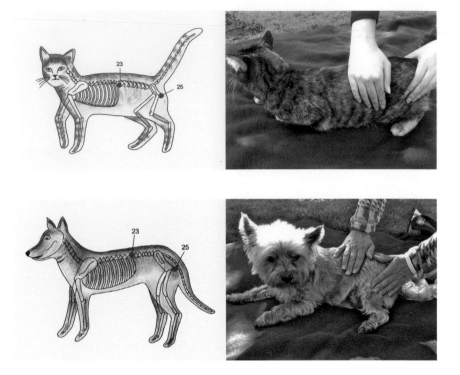

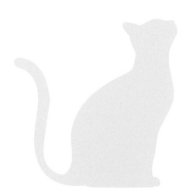

Jin Shin Healing Touch for Cats

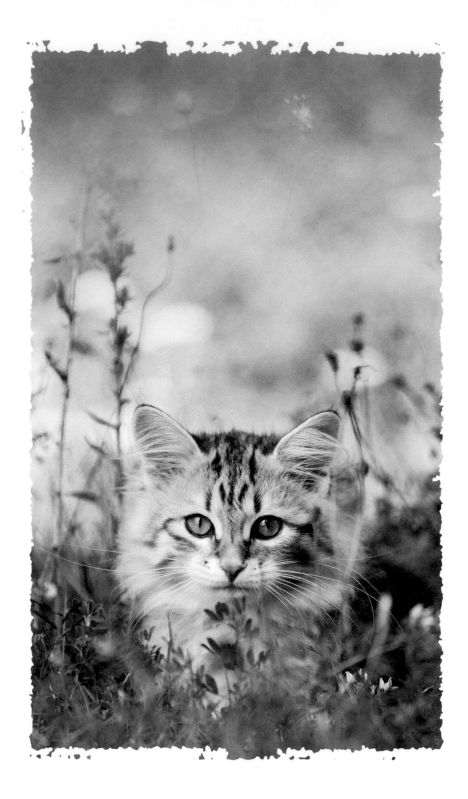

Head

Eyes

Ears

Mouth and Teeth

Brain

EYES

The following hold is good for all eye issues (inflammation, styes, defective vision, etc.) and to fundamentally strengthen the eyes:

> Place one hand on the forehead a little above the affected eye (**SEL 20**) and the other hand on the other side of the body on the neck just below the skull bones (**SEL 4**).

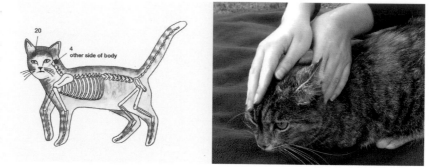

Eye Infection (Conjunctivitis)

The eyelid conjunctiva (connective tissue of the eye) protects the eye. It is very tender and, when healthy, invisible. This mucous membrane can be damaged by dust and grass pollen, and also by strong drafts and the development of bacteria, which can bring about inflammation. Foreign bodies can also be the cause of conjunctivitis – especially if only one eye is affected. Inflammation may also be associated with respiratory infections caused by viruses or bacteria.

> Place one hand on the back of the neck (on both **SELs 4**) and the other hand on the sternum (between both **SELs 13**). Alternatively, use the general eye flow (p. 58).

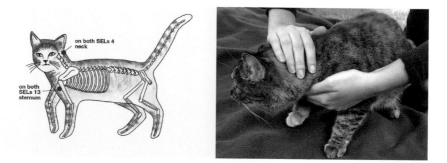

Or place one hand on **SEL 4** on the side of the affected eye and the other hand on **SEL 22** (below the collarbone) on the other side of the body.

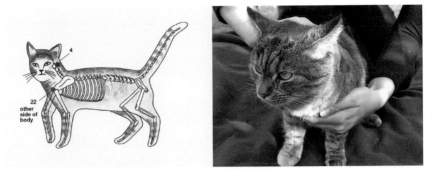

Foreign Objects in the Eye

Place your *left hand* lightly on or slightly above the affected eye and your *right hand* on top of your left. Or hold both **SELs 1** (on the inside of the knee on the hind legs).

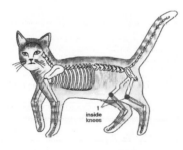
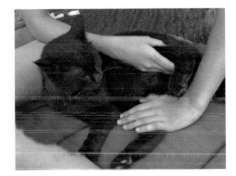

Blocked Tear Ducts

Longer-lasting lacrimation occurring on one or both sides can be due to an obstruction in the tear duct, provided that no change is visible in the outer eye.

To reopen the tear duct, place one hand on the back of the neck between both **SELs 12** and the other hand on the tailbone.

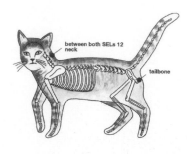 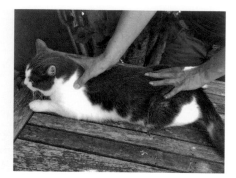

Improving Vision

See info on all eye issues (p. 58 top).

EARS

Hearing

In cases of impaired hearing, place one hand on the neck (on both **SELs 12**) and the other hand on the tailbone (p. 49).

Or hold both **SELs 5** (on the inside ankle of the hind paws).

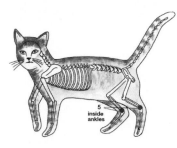 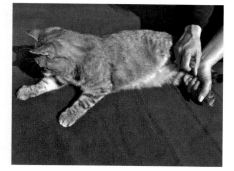

Ear Infection

In ear infections, you can relieve pain by holding the inner and outer bones of the hind paws (**SELs 5** and **SELs 16**).

You can either hold one side of the body and then the other, or you can hold both sides together by holding **SEL 5** and **SEL 16** on the same side with each hand.

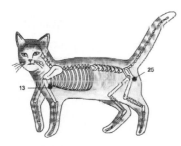
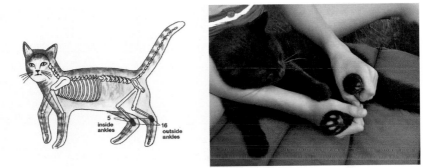

Place one hand on **SEL 13** and the other hand on **SEL 25** on the side of the affected ear.

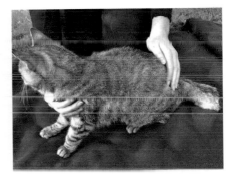
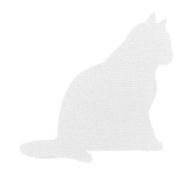

Or place one hand on **SEL 13** and the other hand on **SEL 11**.

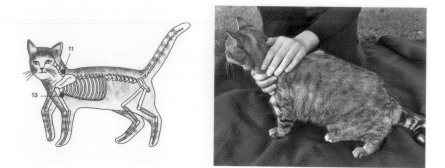

Place your *left hand* on or slightly over the affected ear and your *right hand* on top of your left.

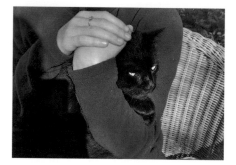

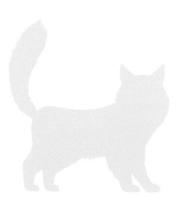

Ear Mites

If your cat repeatedly has ear mites, use the parasite hold:

> Hold both **SELs 19** (in the crook of the elbows) or place one hand on **SEL 19** on the side of the affected ear and the other hand on **SEL 1** on the other side of the body.

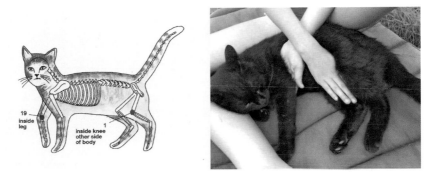

Ear Ulcers

Ear ulcers are often caused by fungi, but can also be caused by an inflammation of the ear canal or by scratch wounds. Use the spleen flow for regular treatments (p. 35). It offers good support for the skin, is used for all fungal diseases and strengthens the immune system.

Ear Hematoma

An ear hematoma is a bruise between the skin and ear cartilage. It is caused by an injury to the edge of the ear, e.g., due to a fight. The affected auricle is warm and marked by swelling. Usually this is not too painful for your pet, but you should still see to it that the bruise disappears soon. You can support this by placing your *right hand* on the affected area and your *left hand* on your *right hand*.

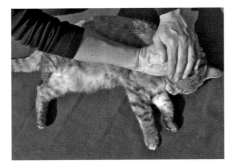

MOUTH AND TEETH

For everything that has to do with the mouth and the teeth, you can use the stomach flow (p. 39) or the quickie for this flow.

Gum Issues

In cases of inflamed gums, or to strengthen the gums, hold **SEL 5** and **SEL 16** with one hand and place the other hand on the calf.

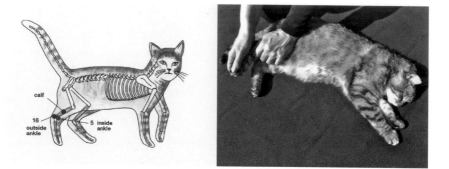

Or apply the first hold of the stomach flow (p. 39).

Inflammation of the Oral Mucous Membrane (Stomatitis)

Frequently an inflammation of the gums and of the oral mucous membrane occurs together for a cat, or rather an inflammation of the oral mucous membrane becomes an issue when an inflammation of the gums spreads.

Triggers are often foreign bodies (fish bones, bone splinters, etc.), the licking of sharp substances, e.g., spices, and the eating of grasses that are infested with mould. Use the holds described under "Gum Issues" (p. 64) and also the spleen flow (p. 35).

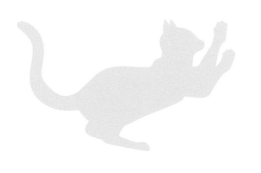

Bad Breath (Halitosis)

An unpleasant smell coming from your cat's mouth can be due to a number of reasons, e.g., diet, stomach or dental issues, gum inflammation, stomatitis or a metabolic disorder. The stomach flow is suitable here (p. 39). It regulates digestion and helps with everything related to the mouth and teeth.

To harmonize the metabolism, hold **SEL 25** together with **SEL 11**.

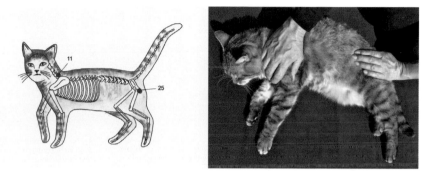

If the symptoms do not improve, have a vet investigate the root cause.

Tumors and Growths

Some cats are predisposed to ulcers on the gum line or the lip. Strengthen the stomach flow (p. 39) as it is the main flow for harmonizing the entire mouth area. The spleen flow (p. 35) supports everything that does not develop harmoniously, especially ulcers, growths, cysts etc.

Hold **SEL 24** together with **SEL 26**.

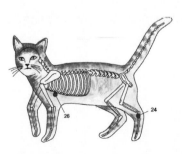
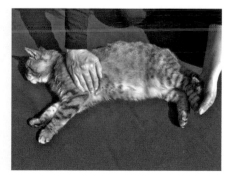

Epilepsy

Epilepsy is a seizure disorder that starts in the brain. Seizures appear as convulsions, muscle spasms or persistent muscle tension and are usually associated with loss of consciousness, changes in behavior and personality, and the loss of urine and feces. This can vary greatly from case to case, depending on the severity of the seizure. Epilepsy can be congenital (although animals usually only become ill from the age of two) or it may occur as a result of other diseases.

In addition to veterinary treatment, you can of course give your cat a lot of support: hold the back paws regularly.

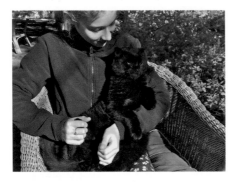

Put one hand on the back of the neck and the other on the forehead.

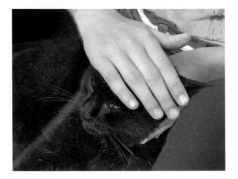

Hold **SEL 12** together with **SEL 14**.

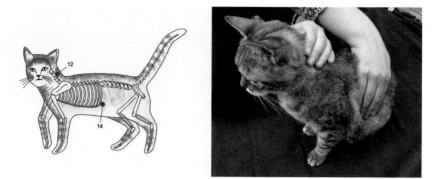

Heart Attack and Cerebral Hemorrhage

These are very rare in cats and when they do occur it is usually in old age. Use the paw flow every day (p. 22).

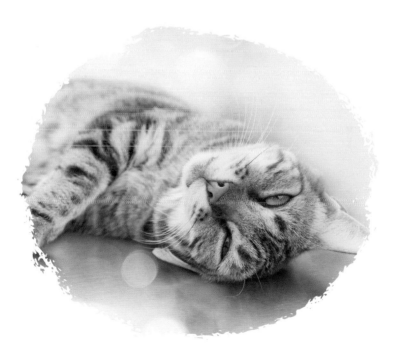

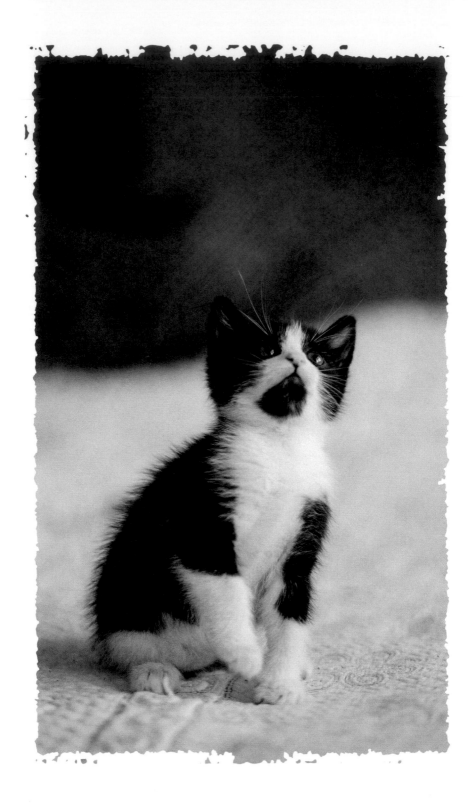

Respiratory System

Cold

Place one hand on **SEL 3** and the other hand on **SEL 11**.

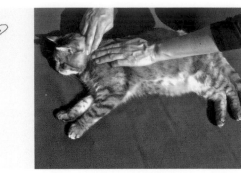

Or hold both **SELs 21**.

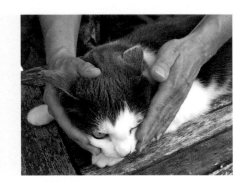

Sinus Infection (Sinusitis)

Hold **SEL 21** and **SEL 22**.

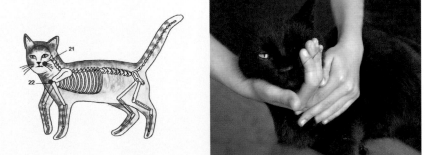

Or place one hand on **SEL 11** and use the other hand to hold the front paw on the other side of the body.

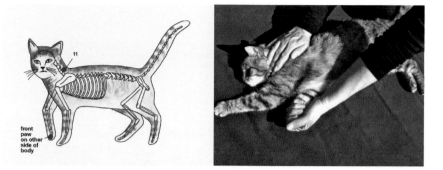

Cat Flu

Cat flu is a collective term for contagious respiratory diseases in cats. It is an infectious disease that primarily causes inflammation of the airways and eyes. Viruses, bacteria or parasites can all be the root cause. The disease occurs in cats all over the world. Young cats with frequent contact with other cats are the most affected (as are cats in animal shelters). Cat flu is especially dangerous for young cats and for those animals with a weakened immune system, and can become chronic or cause permanent damage.

It is important to strengthen the cat's immune system. The main flow for this is the spleen flow (p. 35).

Hold **SEL 3** as often as possible – preferably together with **SEL 15** (p. 89). Also hold **SEL 19** together with high **SEL 19** (about a paw's width above **SEL 19**) by placing one hand on **SEL 19** and the other hand on high **SEL 19** – first on one and then on the other side of the body – or hold **SEL 19** and high **SEL 19** on both sides at the same time.

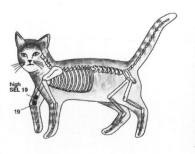
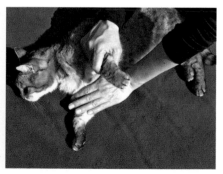

Throat Infection (Laryngitis)

Place one hand on **SEL 11** and **SEL 3** and use the other hand to hold the front paw on the other side of the body.

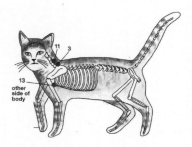
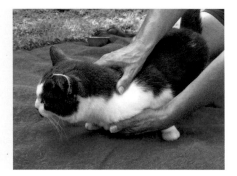

Or place one hand on **SEL 11** and **SEL 3** and the other hand on **SEL 13** on the other side of the body.

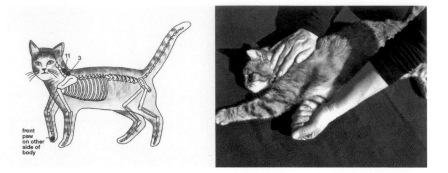

Laryngeal Catarrh

See "Throat Infection (Laryngitis)" (p. 72).

Or place one hand on **SEL 10** and the other hand on **SEL 19**.

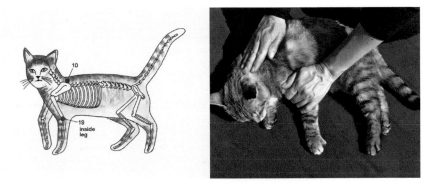

LOWER RESPIRATORY TRACT

Cough and Chest Cold (Bronchitis)

Place one hand on **SEL 10** and the other hand on **SEL 19** (see above).

Or treat **SEL 14** together with **SEL 22**.

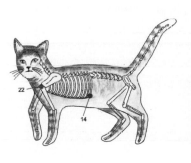 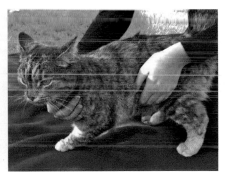

The initial centering hold (p. 20) also helps relieve coughs and chest colds.

Dry Cough

To specifically relieve dry cough, place your hands on the inside of the front legs (slightly diagonally above **SEL 19**).

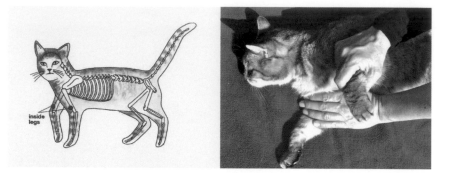

Lung Infection (Pneumonia)

To strengthen the lungs, hold **SEL 14** and **SEL 22** (see above). Or treat **SEL 3** (the so-called antibiotic point) together with **SEL 15** (p. 89).

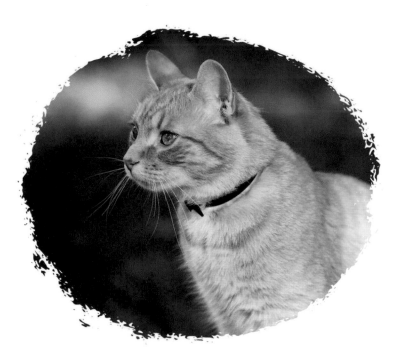

Cardiovascular System

HEART DISEASE AND HEART FAILURE

Fortunately, diseases of the cardiovascular system are rare in cats. If your cat suffers from heart disease, you can offer support (in addition to veterinary treatment).

Hold the left **SEL 15** and the left **SEL 17**.

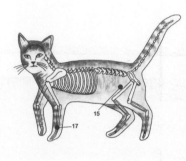 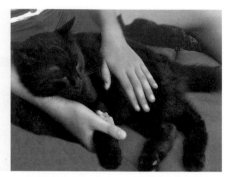

Or hold the left **SEL 11** and left **SEL 17** (front paw joint).

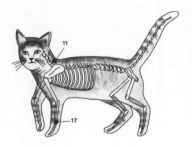 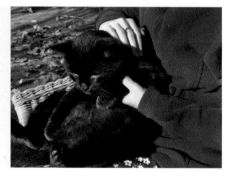

CIRCULATION ISSUES

To strengthen the circulation, e.g., after excessive exertion, collapse or severe diarrhea, hold both **SELs 17**.

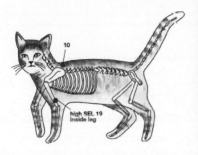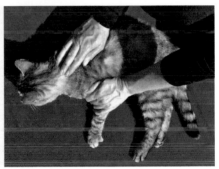

Or put one hand on **SEL 10** and the other hand on high **SEL 19**.

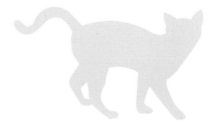

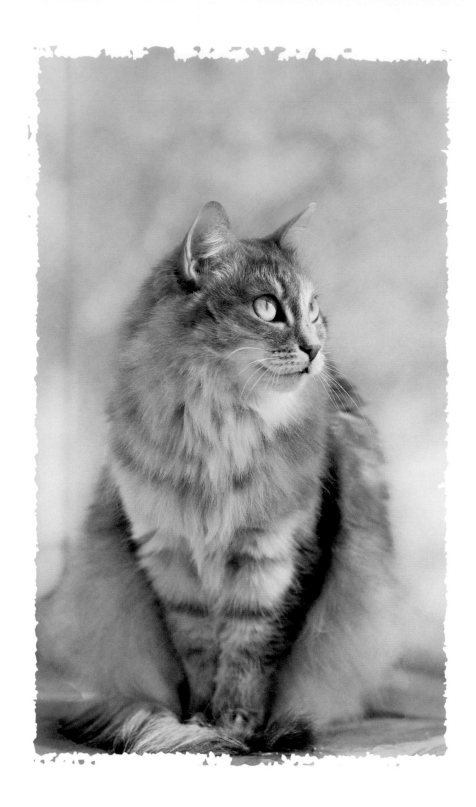

Digestive Organs

STOMACH

The stomach flow is suitable for all issues concerning the stomach (p. 39).

Vomiting

Occasional vomiting to get rid of hairballs or ingested grass is normal. This is how the body eliminates harmful substances. However, if vomiting occurs more frequently, get your cat checked by a vet.

You can also support your cat by holding both **SELs 1**. Or place one hand on **SEL 1** and the other hand on **SEL 14**.

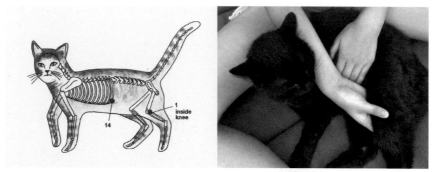

Stomach Pain and Colic

To relieve colic, place your hands on both **SELs 1** (inside knee joints of the hind legs).

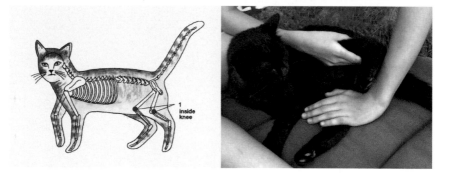

Or hold high **SEL 1** (about one paw's width above **SEL 1**) together with low **SEL 8** (about one paw's width below **SEL 8**).

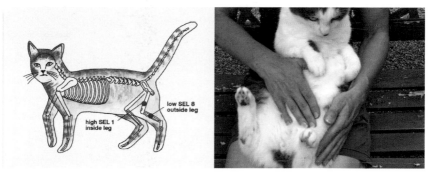

Inflammation of the Stomach Lining (Gastritis)

Gastritis can have different causes: the eating of inedible plants, pollutants in the coat that get into the body from cleaning, drinking of flower water or dishwater, an infection or worm infestation. Gastritis may or may not be accompanied by vomiting.

You can support your cat in the following way: use the stomach flow (p. 39). Hold **SEL 14** and high **SEL 1** on the other side of the body.

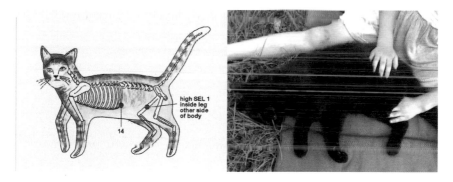

Loss of Appetite

The spleen flow (p. 35) harmonizes eating behavior. It regulates loss of appetite, rejection of food, increased appetite, insatiable appetite etc. The stomach flow (p. 39) also balances appetite and weight.

Weight Loss

The stomach (p. 39) and spleen flows (p. 35) are also suitable in this case. Remember that intestinal parasites (weight loss with normal appetite and eating behavior, p. 83) or thyroid diseases can also be the cause of weight loss.

INTESTINE

Constipation

In cases where there is no evidence of serious illness, constipation may have been caused by a lack of exercise (especially in domestic cats), one-sided diets, food that is too high in fibre and hairballs stuck in the intestine. Make sure your cat always has access to fresh water.

> To clear blockages, hold both **SELs 1** (p. 80). Or place one hand on **SEL 11** and the other hand on the front paw on the other side of the body.

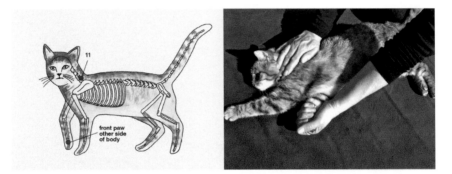

Diarrhea

This can have a number of causes. If it does not improve within a day despite Jin Shin treatment, or if the cat's general condition is impaired, see a vet.

> Hold both **SELs 8**.

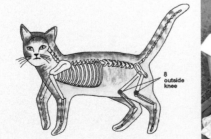
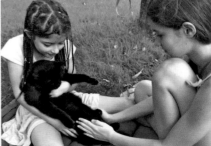

Or place one hand on the right **SEL 8** and the other hand on the right high **SEL 1** (about a paw's width above **SEL 1**).

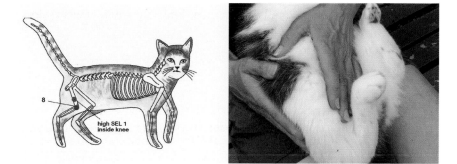

Intestinal Colic

To calm the bowel, you can place one hand on high **SEL 19** and the other hand on **SEL 1** on the other side of the body.

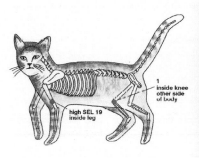
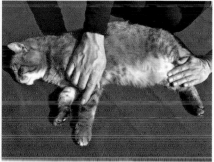

Intestinal Parasites

If your cat has recurring parasite issues, treat both **SELs 19** regularly.

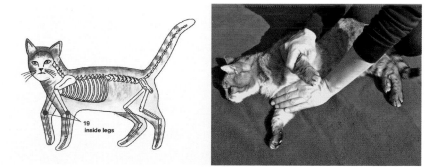

Or hold **SEL 3** together with **SEL 19** first on one side, and then on the other.

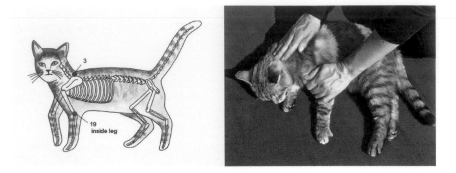

LIVER

The liver is the largest organ of detoxification.

To strengthen the liver, place one hand on the left **SEL 4** and the other hand on the right **SEL 22**.

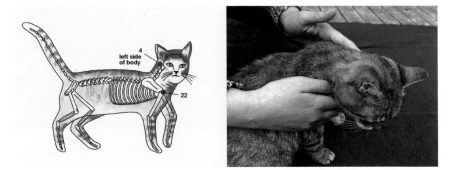

To detox, place one hand on **SEL 12** and the other hand on **SEL 14**.

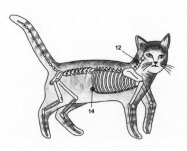
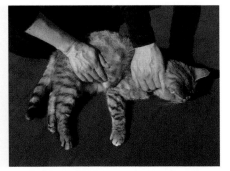

Or treat **SEL 23** together with **SEL 25**.

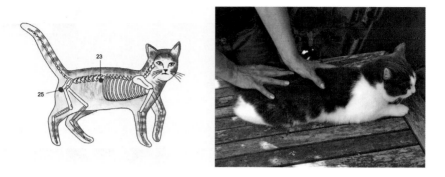

PANCREAS AND SPLEEN

Strengthening the Pancreas

To strengthen the pancreas, hold both **SELs 14**.

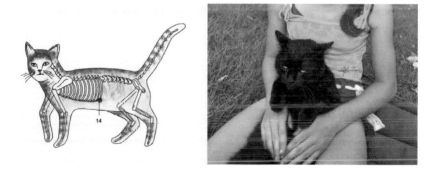

Or place one hand on **SEL 14** and the other hand on high **SEL 1** (about a paw's width above **SEL 1**) on the other side of the body.

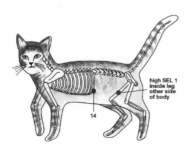 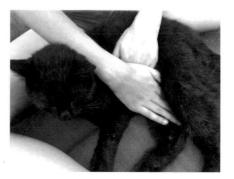

Diabetes

Cats can also have diabetes. In addition to veterinary treatment, you can use the following flow sequence for support:

> **Application for the right side of the body:**
> **STEP 1:** Place your *right hand* on the right **SEL 23** and your *left hand* on the right **SEL 14**.

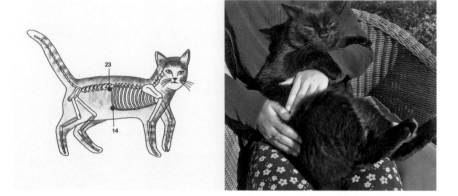

> **STEP 2:** Keep your *right hand* on the right **SEL 23**, and hold the right **SEL 21** with your *left hand*.

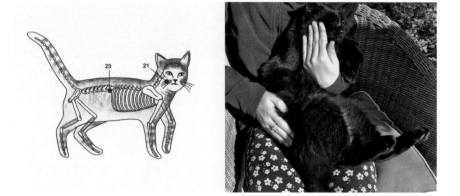

> **And vice versa for the left side of the body:**
> **STEP 1:** *Left hand* on the left **SEL 23**, *right hand* on the left **SEL 14**.
> **STEP 2:** Keep your *left hand* on the left **SEL 23** and move your *right hand* over to the left **SEL 21**.

Urinary System

BLADDER

Bladder Issues

For all bladder issues (inflammation, paralysis etc.), harmonize the bladder flow (p. 48).

Or do the following quickie: place one hand in the middle of the cervical spine between both **SELs 12** and the other hand on the tailbone.

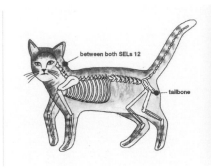 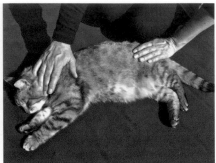

Or treat **SEL 4** together with **SEL 13**.

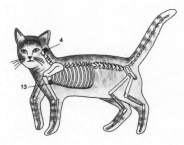 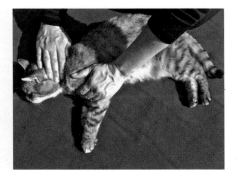

KIDNEYS

Kidney Infection

Application on the right side of the body:

STEP 1: First hold the left **SEL 3** and the left **SEL 15**.

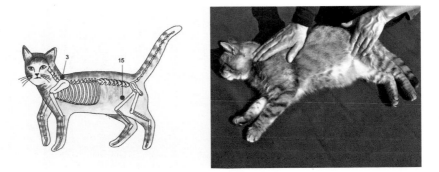

STEP 2: Then place one hand on the pubic bone (in the photo, only the fingertips are used because the cat finds the whole hand uncomfortable). Hold the left hind paw with your other hand.

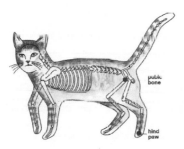
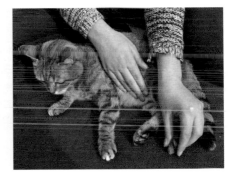

And vice versa for the other side of the body:

STEP 1: One hand on the right **SEL 3** and the other hand on the right **SEL 15**.

STEP 2: One hand on the pubic bone and the other hand on the right hind paw. Or, if your cat does not want to be touched on the pubic bone, place one hand on the back of the neck and the other hand on the tailbone.

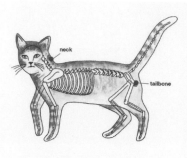 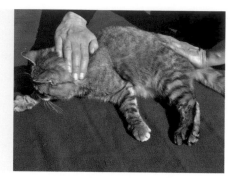

Kidney and Bladder Stones

Hold **SEL 5** and **SEL 16** with one hand and **SEL 23** with the other hand. First do the hold on one side and then on the other side of the body.

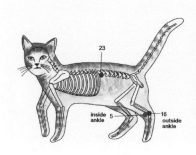 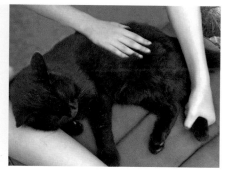

Or treat **SEL 23** together with **SEL 14**.

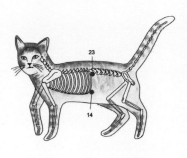

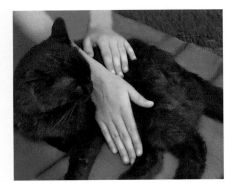

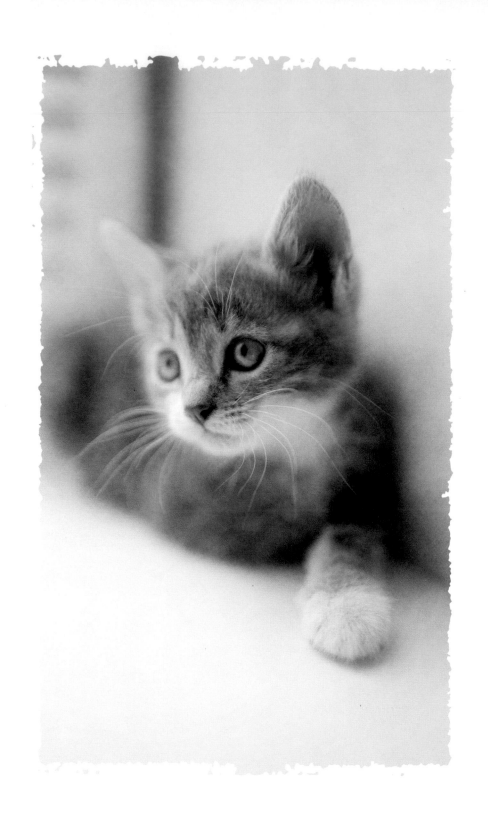

Reproductive Organs

Inflammation of Testes (Testitis)

Hold **SEL 5** together with **SEL 16** with one hand and place the other hand on **SEL 3**.

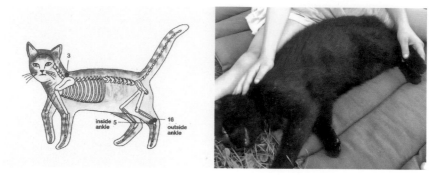

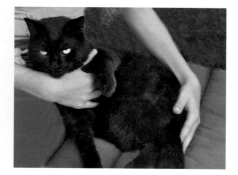

Prostate

Strengthen the spleen flow (p. 31).

Or place one hand on the sternum and the other hand on the tailbone.

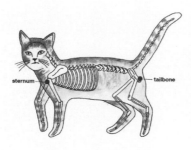

FEMALE REPRODUCTIVE ORGANS
AND BIRTH SUPPORT

Pregnancy

SELs 22 are important for adapting to a new situation (pregnancy, birth and the time afterwards), especially for cats that are giving birth for the first time.

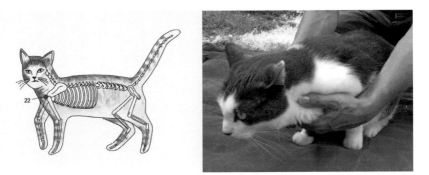

For healthy development during pregnancy, you can regularly use the supervisor flows (p. 35).

SELs 5 held together with SELs 16 supply the uterus with energy.

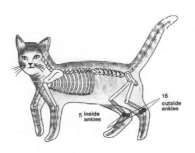

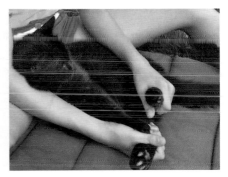

Prenatal Care

SEL 8 softens the pelvis for birth and opens the birth canal. **SEL 22** also prepares the body for birth. You can hold both **SELs** together.

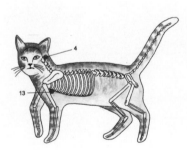
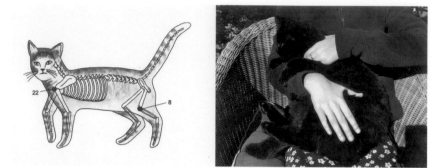

Birth Support

Most cats manage to give birth on their own and most likely will do so in seclusion. There are also cats that seek to be close to their humans. Let the cat do her job. If she turns to you and likes to be touched, you can support her with treatments:

Holding **SEL 13** together with **SEL 4** promotes relaxation and a swift birth.

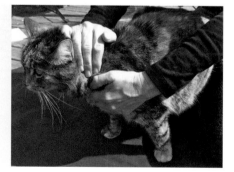

For general birth support and to promote contractions, place one hand on **SEL 8** and the other hand on the sacrum area.

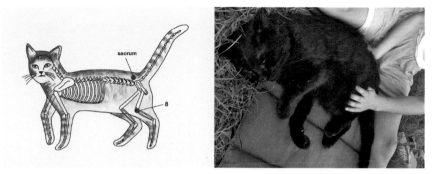

Labour Pains

Treating **SEL 5** together with **SEL 16** relieves pain during the birth.

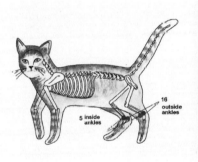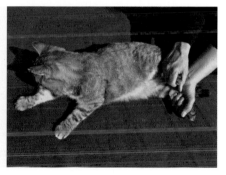

Too Weak or Too Strong Contractions

SEL 1 (p. 124) sets everything into motion and as such promotes the entire birth process. If the delivery stalls, or progresses too quickly, hold **SEL 20** and **SEL 22**.

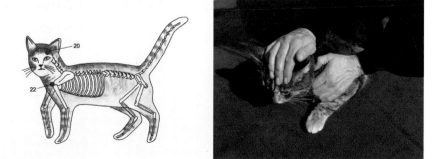

Breathing Issues in Newborn

If a newborn kitten is having difficulty breathing, hold both **SELs 4**.

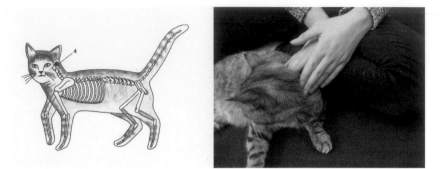

Milk Shortage or Surplus

Milk flow usually regulates itself. If this is not the case, you can support your cat by using the spleen flow (p. 35).

Or place one hand on **SEL 22** and the other hand on **SEL 14**.

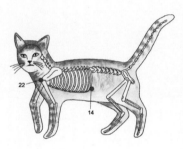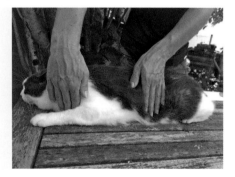

Inflammation of Teats

First place one hand on **SEL 3** and the other hand on **SEL 15** (p. 89). Then treat high **SEL 19** (approximately one paw's width above **SEL 19**) together with high **SEL 1** (approximately one paw's width above **SEL 1**) on the other side of the body.

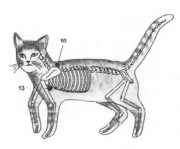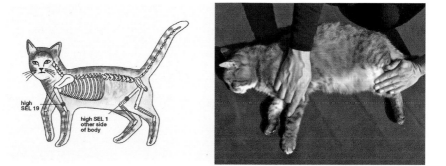

Pseudo-Pregnancy

Hold **SEL 10** and **SEL 13** first on one side and then on the other side of the body.

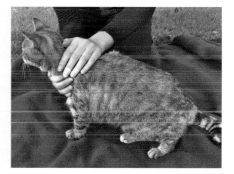

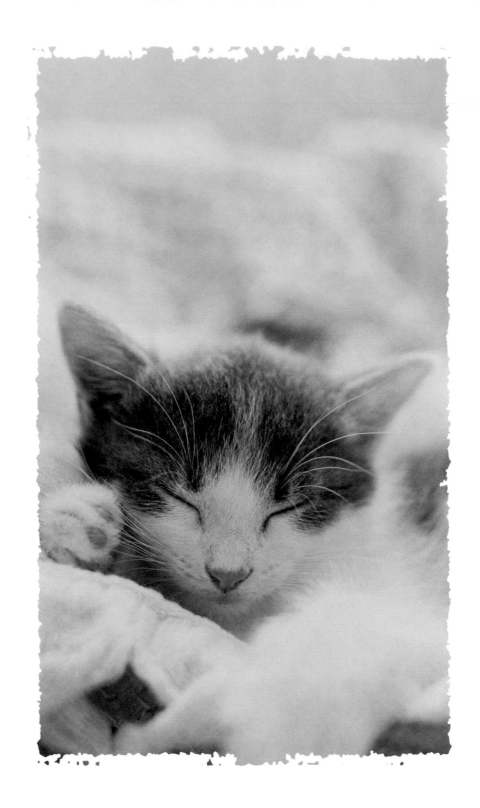

Coat and Skin

The stomach flow (p. 39) is the skin and hair specialist. If your cat has skin or coat issues, it is a good idea to use this flow regularly. Also, pay attention to a healthy and balanced diet.

COAT

Hair Loss

In addition to the stomach flow (p. 39), also treat **SEL 14** together with **SEL 22** on the other side of the body.

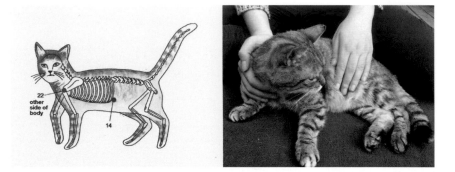

Other possible causes of hair loss are chronic organ diseases, parasites, fungal or hormonal disorders. Always have the cause clarified by a vet.

Dull Coat

Use the spleen flow regularly (p. 35).

Dandruff

Harmonize the stomach (p. 39) and spleen flows (p. 35).

SKIN

Eczema

Regularly treat **SEL 3** together with **SEL 19**.

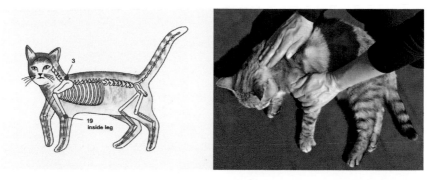

Or hold **SEL 14** together with **SEL 22**.

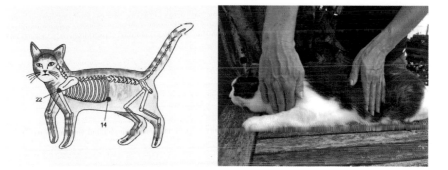

Boils and Abscesses

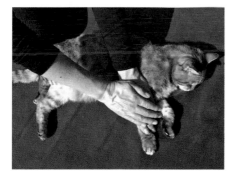

For boils and abscesses, place your *left hand* on the abscess and your *right hand* on top of the *left hand*.

If you are in the company of others, you can also create a "mountain of hands":

> Place your *left hand* on the abscess and the **right hand** on the *left hand*; the next person places their *left hand* on your *right hand* and their **right hand** on their *left hand* etc. This speeds up the healing process.

Itching

To relieve itching, hold **SEL 3** together with **SEL 4**.

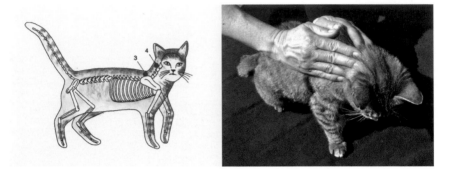

Fungal Skin Infection

The spleen flow (p. 35) supports all fungal diseases.

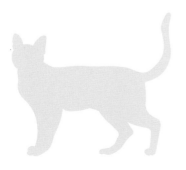

Allergies and Intolerances

Allergies and intolerances are nowadays not only a common issue for humans, but also for cats. There are different factors that can trigger an allergy, and often we can only guess at what the root cause may be. In allergies, the immune system is fighting substances that it should not be fighting. Therefore, harmonizing the immune system is essential in treating all allergies.

SEL 3 is the key to an intact immune system. It is, so to speak, the door that swings open so that viruses and bacteria can leave the body again and through which the body can receive new, purified energy.

Hold **SEL 3** together with **SEL 15**.

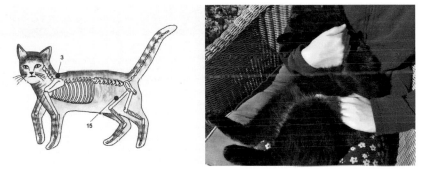

The spleen flow (p. 35) also strengthens the immune system. Another important hold for allergies is the following:

Place one hand on **SEL 19** and the other hand on **SEL 1**.

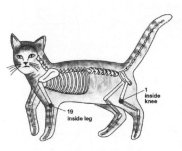
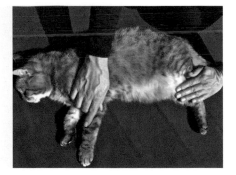

An essential SEL for all intolerances is **SEL 22**. Hold **SEL 22** together with **SEL 14**.

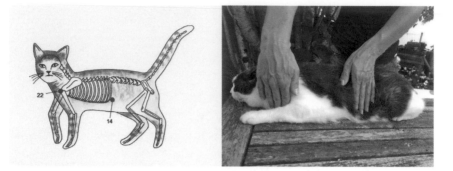

The hold for initial centering is also very helpful (p. 20).

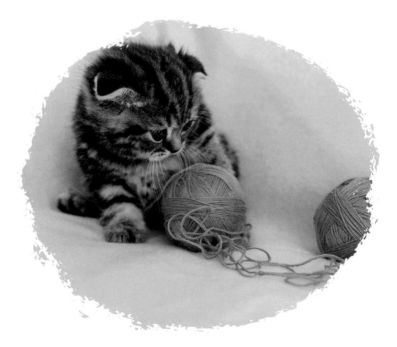

Nervous System

MUSCLE TWITCHING

Muscle twitching can be an accompanying symptom of various neurological diseases, e.g., disturbances in the nervous system and in the nerve cells of the muscles. Have this checked out by a vet.

However, there is not always a disease behind muscle twitching. It is often harmless. Sometimes the symptom is also due to temporary nerve irritation. Hold **SEL 8** together with **SEL 17**.

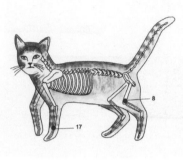
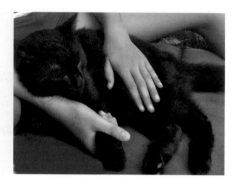

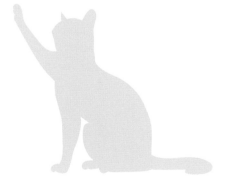

PARALYSIS

In cases of paralysis, use the following holds in sequence:

For the right side of the body:

STEP 1: Place your *left hand* on the right **SEL 4** and your *right hand* on the right **SEL 13**.

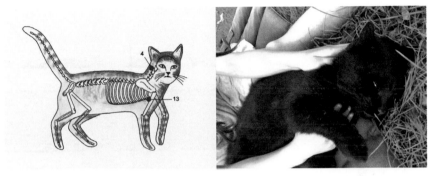

STEP 2: Then place your *right hand* on the right **SEL 16** and your *left hand* on the right **SEL 15**.

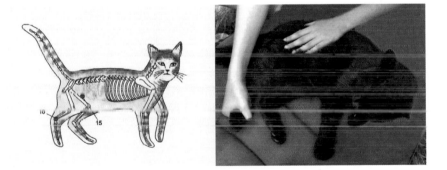

For the left side of the body, reverse the holds:

STEP 1: Place your *right hand* on the left **SEL 4** and the *left hand* on the left **SEL 13**.

STEP 2: Then place your *left hand* on top of your left **SEL 16** and the *right hand* on the left **SEL 15**.

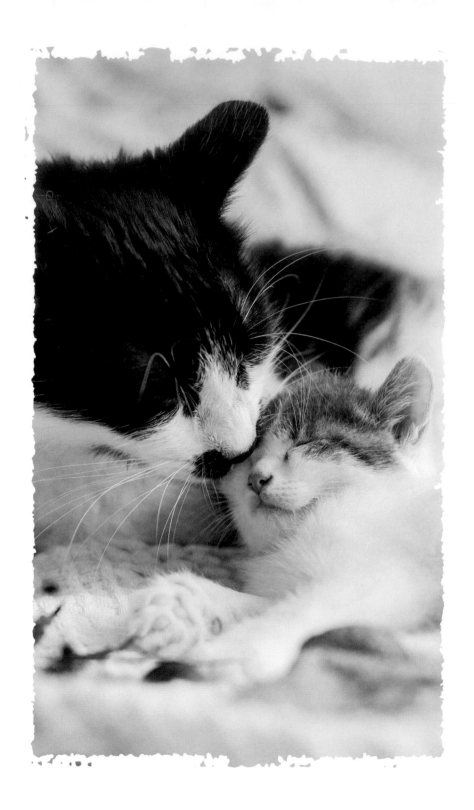

Musculoskeletal System

BACK AND SPINE

The so-called chiropractor flow involves the following hold:

Place one hand on **SEL 2** and hold first one and then the other hind paw with the other hand.

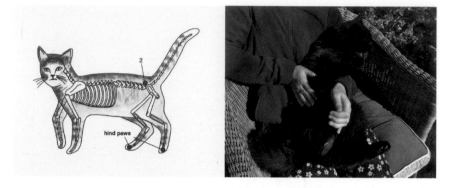

An important flow for everything to do with the back is the bladder flow (p. 48). The paw flow (p. 22) also harmonizes the back and intervertebral discs.

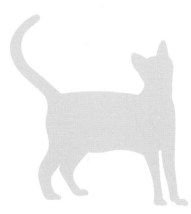

MUSCLES

The following holds support the muscles and help with muscle inflammation, strains, overexertion, tremors, too high or too low muscle tone and muscle pain:

Place one hand on **SEL 8**, and with the other hand hold **SEL 5** together with **SEL 16**.

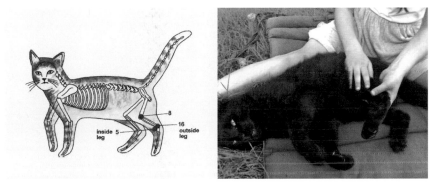

Muscle Cramps

Hold both **SELs 8** or **SEL 8** together with **SEL 1** on the other side of the body.

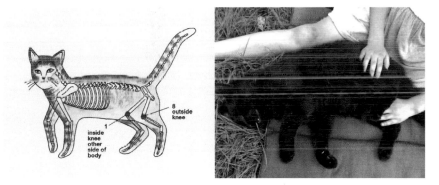

LIGAMENTS, TENDONS, AND JOINTS

Sprains and Strains

If the front paw is sprained, hold the affected joint.

If the hind paw is sprained, hold the front leg on the other side of the body by the first joint and with the other hand hold **SEL 15** on the same side as the front leg.

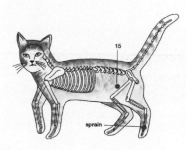
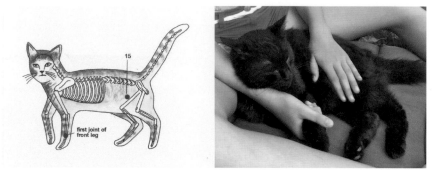

Or place one hand on the affected area and the other hand on **SEL 15** on the same side of the body.

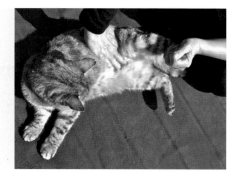

Strengthening Ligaments and Tendons

To strengthen ligaments and tendons, place one hand on **SEL 4** and the other hand on **SEL 22**.

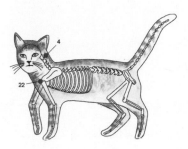
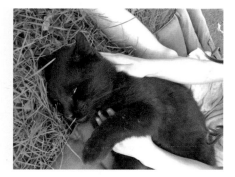

Joint Inflammation (Arthritis)

Place one hand on **SEL 12** and the other hand on **SEL 14**.

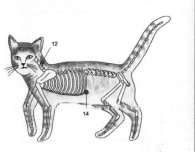
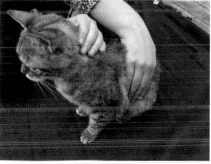

To relieve pain and heal the inflammation, hold **SEL 5** and **SEL 16** with one hand and **SEL 3** with the other hand.

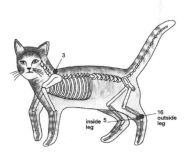
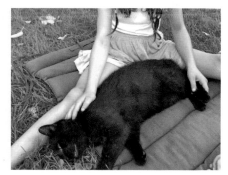

Joint Abrasion (Osteoarthritis)

Hold **SEL 13** and **SEL 17**.

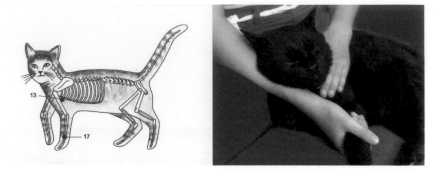

Treating **SEL 1** brings movement and mobility. Hold both **SELs 1** (p. 59) or **SEL 1** together with high **SEL 19** (approximately a paw's width above **SEL 19**).

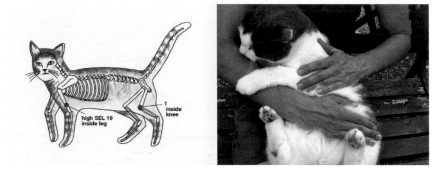

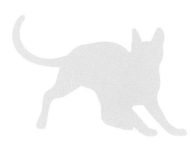

BONES

Broken Bones

Hold **SEL 15** to support healing in broken bones. To do so, place both hands in the groin. You can also treat **SEL 15** together with **SEL 3**.

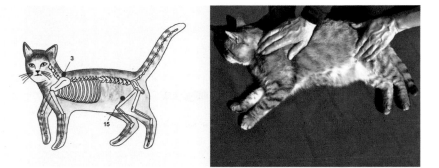

Strengthening Bones

To strengthen the bones, hold **SEL 13** together with **SEL 11** on the opposite side of the body.

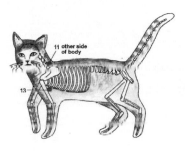
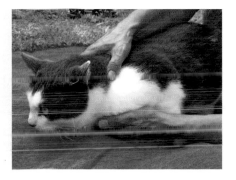

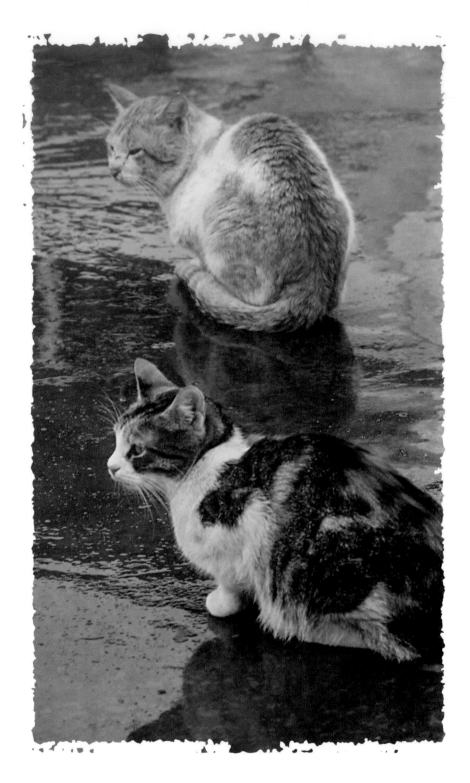

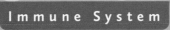

Immune System

IMMUNE SYSTEM

An intact immune system is a prerequisite for health and vitality. As soon as you treat your cat, you automatically strengthen its immune system and stimulate its self-healing powers. The most important SEL for a well-functioning immune system is **SEL 3**. When **SEL 3** is in harmony, bacteria and viruses, which are in actual fact always present in the body, can leave the body again without getting stuck and triggering diseases. You can also stop and dissolve incipient infections by holding **SEL 3** together with **SEL 15** (p. 89).

Further flows can harmonize the immune system very effectively and powerfully:

- the main central flow (p. 22)
- the supervisor flows (p. 31)
- the spleen flow (p. 35)

Or hold **SEL 19** together with high **SEL 19**.

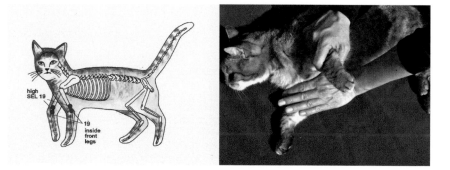

Infectious Diseases

INFECTIOUS DISEASES

If your cat has an infectious disease such as the feline parvovirus, leukemia virus, immunodeficiency virus or feline infectious peritonitis, then it definitely belongs in the hands of a vet.

As a preventive measure, you can support your cat's immune system (p. 120) with treatments so as to give it the chance to deal with all adversities in the best possible way.

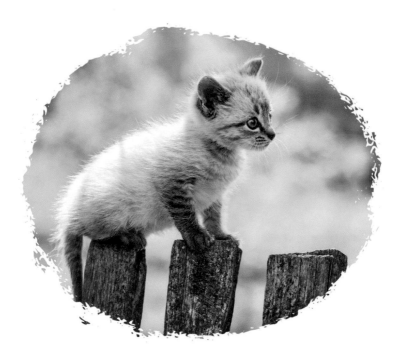

Edema, Growths, and Tumors

To dissolve edema, apply the bladder flow (p. 48).

GROWTHS AND TUMORS

Where there is movement, no accumulation can build up. Treatments bring the flow of energy back into motion, so that whatever is old and hardened can be loosened. Jin Shin Jyutsu harmonizes the whole being and gradually brings everything back into balance – including cell growth.

SEL 1, the original mover, sets everything into motion and dissolves accumulations.

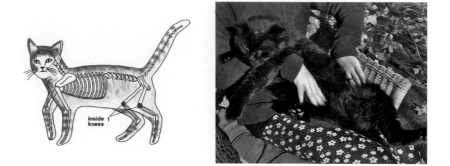

The spleen flow (p. 35) brings light into every cell and can dissolve tumors and accumulations. Apply the main central flow (p. 22) regularly.

To support cell renewal, hold **SEL 20** and the back of **SEL 19** on the other side of the body.

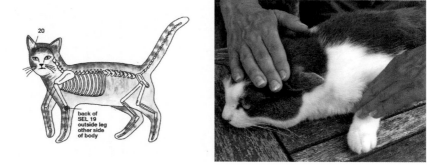

Use the supervisor flows regularly (p. 31).

An important hold for malignant tumors is the following:

Place one hand on **SEL 24** (harmonizes chaos) and the other hand on **SEL 26**. This is also an effective hold for cysts.

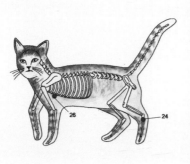
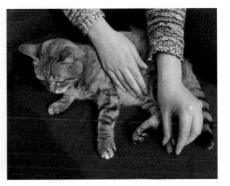

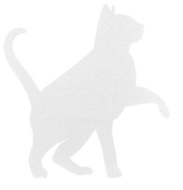

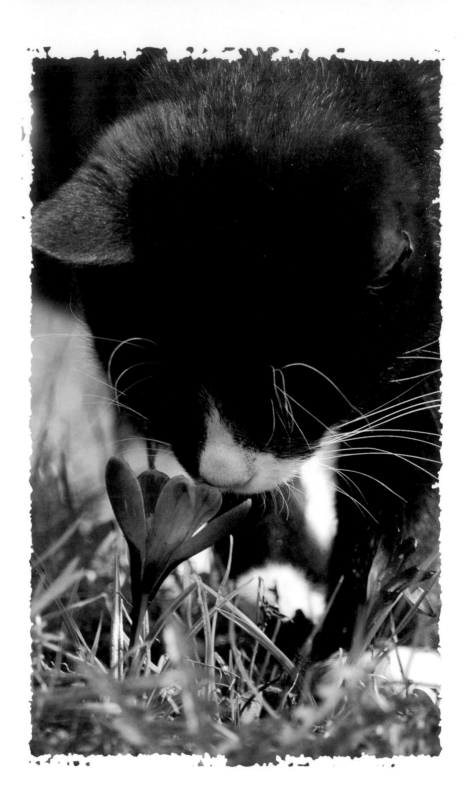

Behavior and Psyche

FEAR AND PANIC

An important flow for fear is the main central flow (p. 22). It brings everything back to the center and evokes deep trust.

Place one hand in the area of both **SELs 4**, **12** and **11** (behind the neck) and the other hand on both **SELs 22** (under the collarbones).

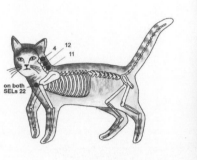
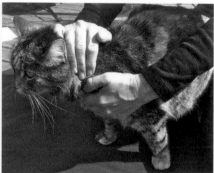

INSECURITIES AND NERVOUSNESS

For all insecure or nervous cats, regularly apply the main central flow (p. 22) and hold both **SELs 17** together with both **SELs 18**.

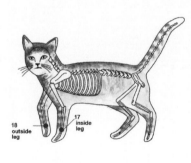
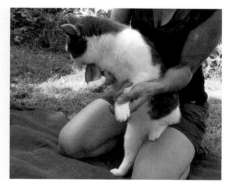

STARTLE RESPONSES

The main central flow helps here too (p. 22).

Or place one hand on **SEL 23** and the other hand on **SEL 26**.

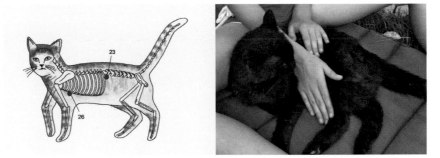

FOOD ENVY

Hold **SEL 14** and high **SEL 19** (about a paw's width above **SEL 19**).

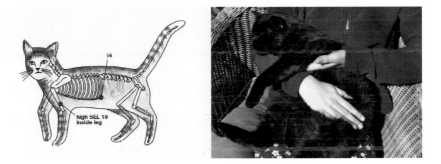

FIGHTING AND AGGRESSION

If your cat is frequently involved in fights, ensure good basic harmonizing treatments, e.g., through the main central flow (p. 22).

Hold **SEL 24** together with **SEL 26**.

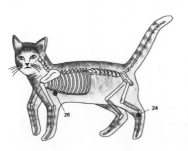
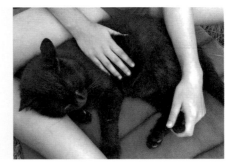

Place one hand on both **SELs 4** (behind the neck) and the other hand on both **SELs 22** (under the collarbones).

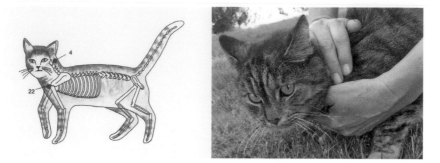

NEGLECT AND ABUSE

If your cat has been neglected in its previous home, you can balance this disharmony with the spleen flow (p. 35).

The hold for initial centering (p. 20) helps the cat to gradually process negative experiences.

SENSITIVITY TO NOISE

If your cat is very sensitive to noise, use one hand to hold **SEL 22** together with **SEL 13**, and put the other hand on **SEL 17**.

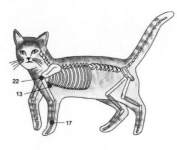
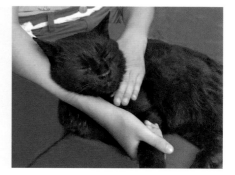

The spleen flow (p. 35) also helps with hypersensitivities of all kinds.

Injuries and Emergencies

Bleeding Wounds

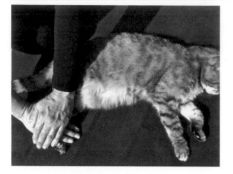

Place your *right hand* on top of or slightly over the wound or dressing and your *left hand* on top of your *right hand*.
Placing the *right hand* first helps to retain whatever should remain in the body.

Festering Wounds

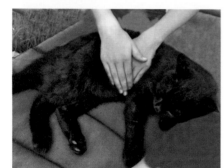

Place your *left hand* on or over the wound and your *right hand* on top of your *left hand*.
Placing the *left hand* first helps to extract whatever needs to leave the body.

IMPORTANT: Do not worry about confusing left and right and thereby causing exactly the opposite of what you intended to happen. Treatments are always linked to the intelligence of the body. If, for example, you mix up your hands, the body turns this around by itself – it may take a little longer for the effect to set in, but nothing else will happen.

STINGS, SPLINTERS, AND THORNS

Place your *left hand* on or over the affected area and your *right hand* on top of your *left hand*.

BURNS

Place both hands next to each other on or over the affected area.

CONCUSSION

First hold both **SELs 4**.

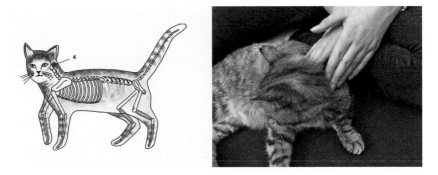

Then hold both hind paws.

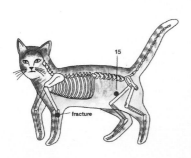

BROKEN BONES

Place your hands on both **SELs 15**, or place one hand on the fractured bone and the other hand on **SEL 15** on the same side of the body.

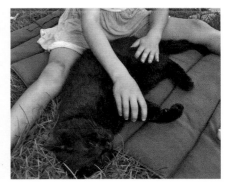

BRUISES

Place your *right hand* on the affected area and your *left hand* on your *right hand*.

SHOCK

Shock is a life-threatening affliction of the circulatory system. An affected animal definitely belongs in the hands of a vet! Shock can be caused by a number of things, e.g., heatstroke, injuries with severe blood loss, fights, poisoning, allergies, accidents etc. A shocked cat is usually calm, it breathes quickly and shallowly, and its pulse is accelerated and weak. The usually pink mucous membranes are very pale and the cat feels cool.

Take the cat to the vet and treat both **SELs 1** with your hands crossed.

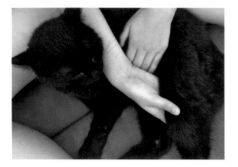

POISONING

In the event of poisoning, a vet must be consulted immediately.

As first aid, hold both **SELs 1** with your hands crossed (see above). Also hold **SEL 21** and **SEL 23**.

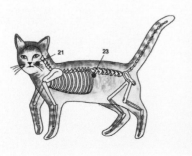

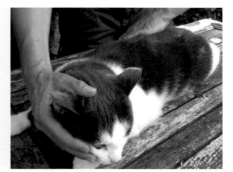

HEATSTROKE AND SUNSTROKE

Important: never cool a cat down too quickly! Take it to a shady place and moisten its coat with a cloth. Offer it water or drip a little onto its tongue. The first aid hold for too much sun or heat is:

Hold both **SELs 4** (p. 133). Then hold both **SELs 7** (p. 17).

CHOKING AND SHORTNESS OF BREATH

Hold both **SELs 1** or **SEL 1** together with **SEL 2**.

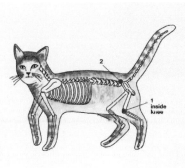 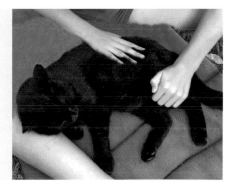

OPERATIONS

Hold both **SELs 15** before and after operations.

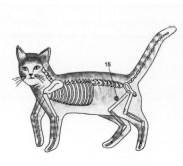 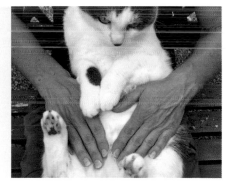

PAIN

You can relieve all kinds of pain by holding **SEL 5** together with **SEL 16**.

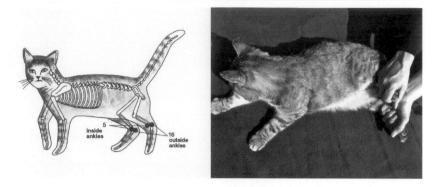

END-OF-LIFE CARE

If your cat is dying, you can hold **SEL 4** with **SEL 13** to ease its transition.

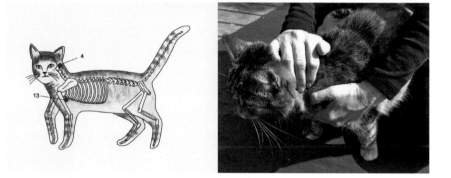

SEL 4 is an important SEL for all transitions. It is said that it stops from dying those whose time has not yet come, and it helps those who have reached the end of their life to pass over.

Other Issues

HOUSE-TRAINING

Apply the bladder flow (p. 48).

LACK OF CLEANLINESS

If your cat is a little careless with grooming itself, place one hand on the back of the neck on both **SELs 12** and the other hand on the tailbone (base of the tail).

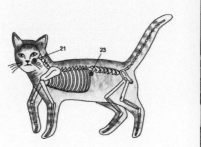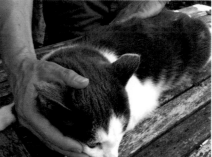

HARMONIZING SIDE EFFECTS OF MEDICATION

To harmonize the side effects of drugs, treat **SEL 21** and **SEL 23** first on one side and then on the other side of the body.

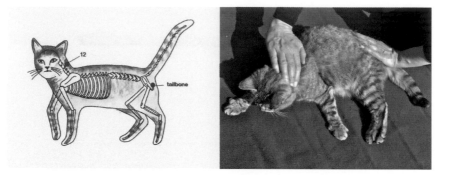

Hold both **SELs 22** or **SEL 22** together with **SEL 23**.

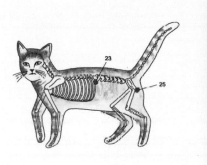 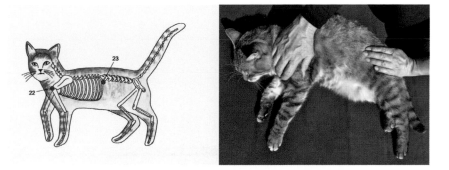

ALLEVIATING REACTIONS TO VACCINES

Apply the spleen flow (p. 35) or treat **SEL 23** and **SEL 25**.

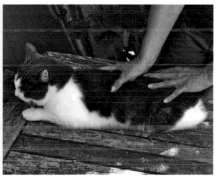 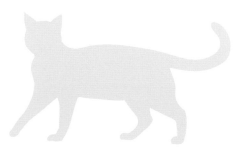

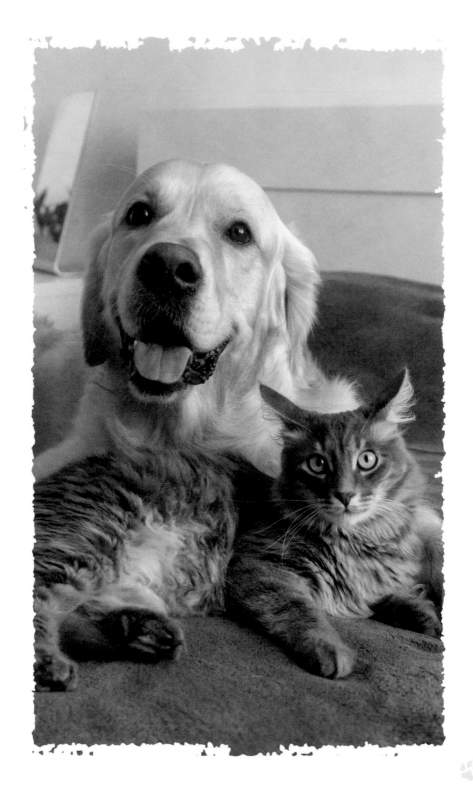

Jin Shin Healing
Touch for Dogs

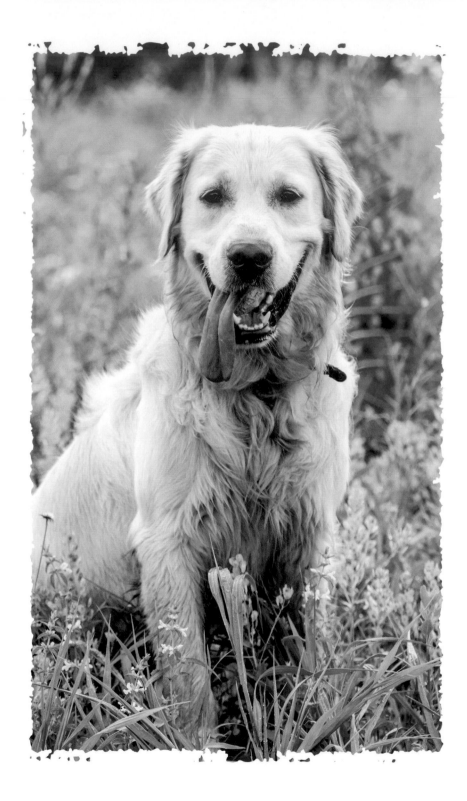

Head

EYES

The following hold is good for all eye issues (eye inflammation, styes, defective vision etc.) or for a general strengthening of the eyes:

> Place one hand on the forehead a little above the affected eye (**SEL 20**) and the other hand on the other side of the body on the neck just below the skull bone (**SEL 4**).

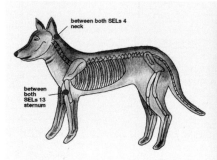
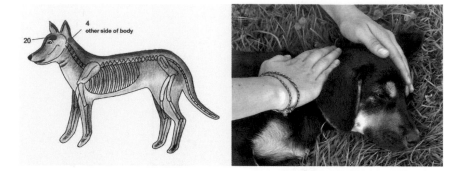

Improving Vision

> In addition to the aforementioned hold, you can also place one hand on the neck (between both **SELs 4**) and the other hand on the breastbone (**SEL 13**).

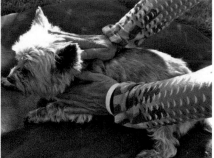

Place one hand under the collarbone on the side of the affected eye (**SEL 22**) and the other hand on the other side of the body on the neck below the skull bone (**SEL 4**).

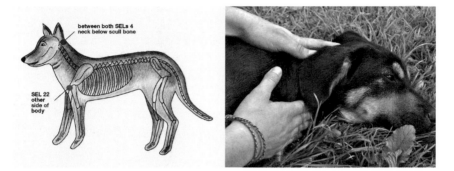

Eye Infection (Conjunctivitis)

See the general hold for all eye issues (p. 144 top).

Foreign Objects in the Eye

Place your *left hand* lightly on or slightly above the affected eye and your *right hand* on top of your *left hand*. Or hold both **SELs 1** (inside knee of hind legs).

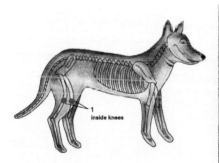
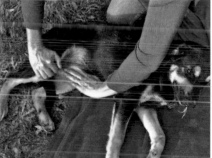

Blocked Tear Ducts

When there is no change visible on the outer eye, long-term lacrimation occurring on one or both sides can be due to an obstruction in the tear duct.

> To open the tear duct again, place one hand on the back of the neck between both **SELs 12** and the other hand on the tailbone.

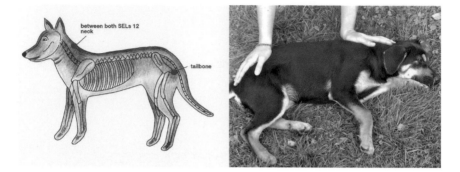

Nictitating Membrane Issues

Some dog breeds with thick hanging lips, e.g., Great Danes or boxers, often suffer from an inversion of the nictitating cartilage or from swollen nictitating glands, which then often leads to conjunctivitis. This is due to slack connective tissue in the area around the eyes.

> The following hold helps to strengthen the connective tissue: place one hand on the outside of the ankle on the hind leg (**SEL 16**) and the other hand on the buttocks below the seat-bone (**SEL 25**) – both on the affected side of the body.

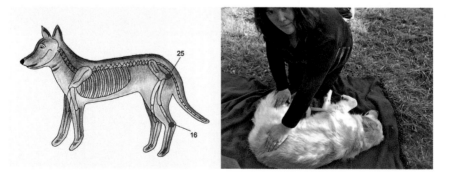

EARS

The bladder flow (p. 48) has a supportive and harmonizing effect on everything that has to do with the ears and hearing.

As a quickie, you can put one hand on the neck (between both **SELs 12**) and the other hand on the tailbone.

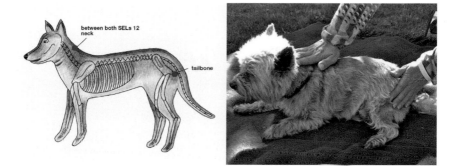

Hearing

If hearing is impaired, you can hold both **SELs 5** (inner ankle on hind paws) in addition to the aforementioned holds.

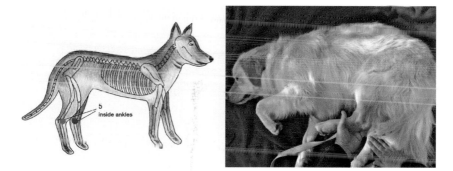

Or you can place one hand on the pubic bone and the other hand in the area of the little toe of the hind paw on the side of the affected ear.

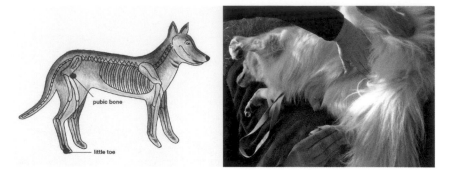

Ear Infection

For ear infections, hold the inner and outer ankles of the hind leg to relieve the pain (**SEL 5** and **SEL 16**). You can either treat one side of the body and then the other, or you can treat both sides together by holding each **SEL 5** and **SEL 16** with one hand.

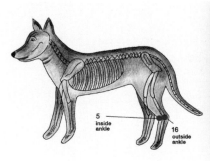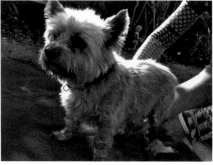

Place one hand on **SEL 13** and the other hand on **SEL 25** on the side of the affected ear.

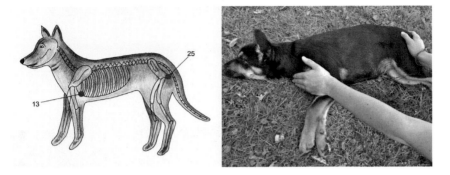

Place your *left hand* on or slightly over the affected ear and your *right hand* on top of your *left hand*.

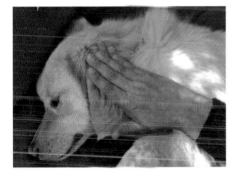

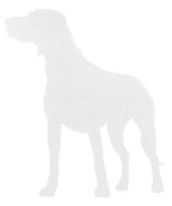

Ear Mites

If your dog has ear mites repeatedly, use the parasite hold: hold both **SELs 19** (in the crook of the elbows) or place one hand on **SEL 19** on the side of the affected ear and the other hand on **SEL 1** on the other side of the body.

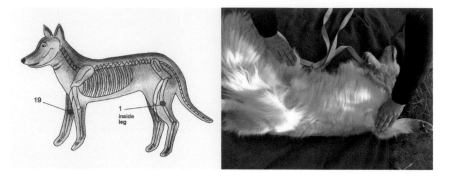

Auricular Eczema

Auricular eczema, which is usually chronic, can be harmonized well with the spleen flow (p. 35). The spleen flow is a good support for the skin and is the flow of choice for all fungal diseases. Very often auricular eczema also involves fungal cells.

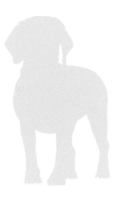

MOUTH AND TEETH

The stomach flow (p. 39) or the shortcut for it, if you find the flow itself is too long for you, is suitable for everything that has to do with the mouth and teeth.

Teething

Not only babies, but also puppies can have a hard time when their milk teeth are replaced by permanent teeth.

> First, place one hand on **SEL 5** and **SEL 16** and the other hand on the calf. Then continue to hold **SEL 5** and **SEL 16** with one hand and place the other hand on the tailbone.

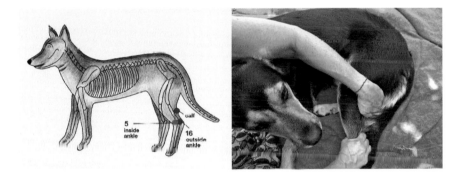

For small dogs, you can hold **SEL 16** and the calf together and **SEL 25** with the other hand.

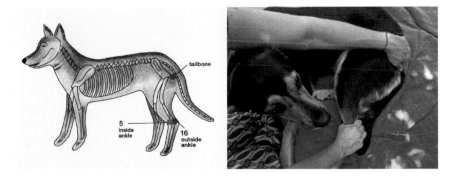

Tooth Decay

Dogs are even less fond of going to the dentist than humans, so it is very important to prevent tooth decay. A healthy diet is important for this. Do not give your dog candy, cake, or anything else off the table. Healthy chewing products for canine dental care are available in specialist shops.

> For preventative treatment for tooth decay: use the stomach flow regularly (p. 39). Or hold **SEL 16** together with low **SEL 8** (about a paw's width below **SEL 8**).

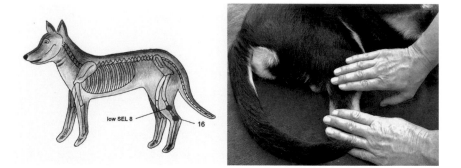

Gum Issues

> If the gums are inflamed or to strengthen the gums, hold **SEL 5** and **SEL 16** with one hand and place the other hand on low **SEL 8**.

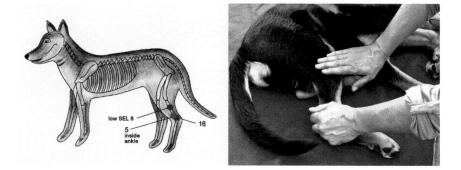

> Or use the first hold of the stomach flow (p. 39).

Bad Breath (Halitosis)

An unpleasant smell coming from your dog's snout can have different causes, e.g., incorrect feeding, stomach issues, dental issues, pelvic eczema or a metabolic disorder.

The stomach flow is suitable here (p. 39). It regulates digestion and supports everything that has to do with the mouth and teeth.

To harmonize the metabolism, hold **SEL 25** together with **SEL 11**.

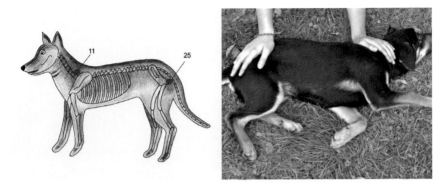

Lip Fold Eczema (Dermatitis)

In lip fold eczema or lip fold dermatitis, bacteria and fungi accumulate in the skin folds of the lips and trigger inflammation, which becomes noticeable through an extremely unpleasant odour. Take good care of the skin folds. Clean them after eating, and always keep the food bowl clean, as this quickly gathers bacteria, which can then trigger an inflammation in the dog.

Hold **SEL 3** for the inflammation, preferably together with **SEL 15**.

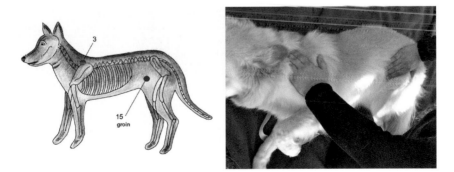

Mouth Rot (Infectious Stomatitis)

Use the stomach flow (p. 39) or the quickie for it.

BRAIN

Meningitis

Meningitis is not to be trifled with. It is a serious life-threatening disease.

You can, however, accompany medical treatment with Jin Shin Jyutsu flows: hold **SEL 5** and **SEL 16** with one hand and **SEL 7** with the other hand.

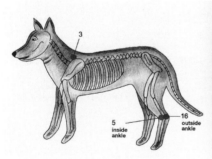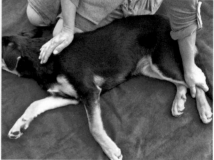

Then place the hand that is on **SEL 7** on **SEL 3**. Do the holds first on one side of the body and then on the other side.

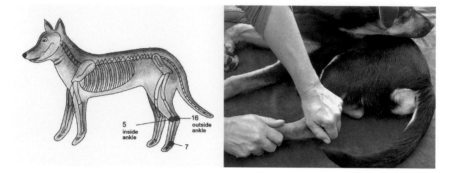

Stroke

Use the paw flow daily (p. 22). For supportive treatment after a stroke hold **SEL 7** or **SEL 7** together with **SEL 6** as often as possible.

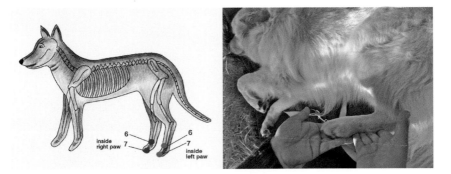

On the side opposite the affected one, hold the **SELs** in the following order: **SEL 5** and **SEL 16**.

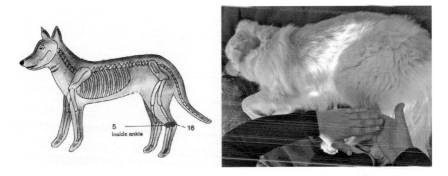

SELs 5 and **SEL 15**

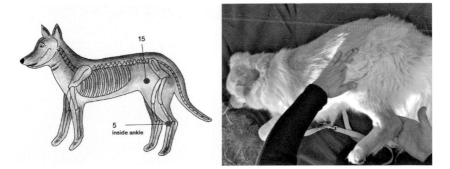

SEL 5 and SEL 23

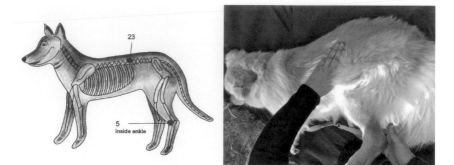

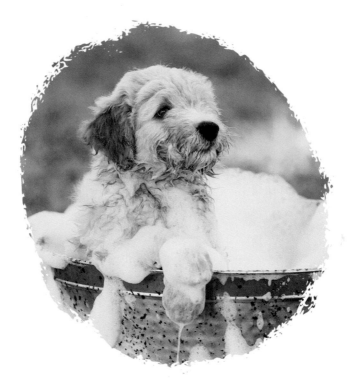

Respiratory System

UPPER RESPIRATORY TRACT

Cold

Place one hand on **SEL 3** and the other hand on **SEL 11**.

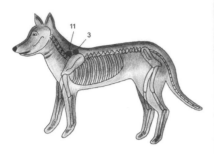
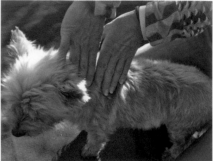

Or hold both **SELs 21**.

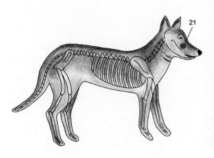
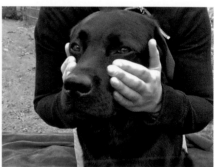

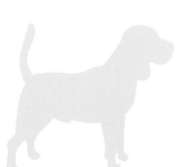

Sinus Infection (Sinusitis)

Hold **SEL 21** together with **SEL 22**.

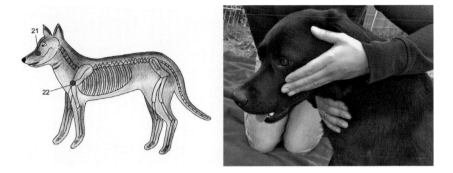

Or place one hand on **SEL 11** and with the other hand hold the second toe of the front paw on the other side of the body.

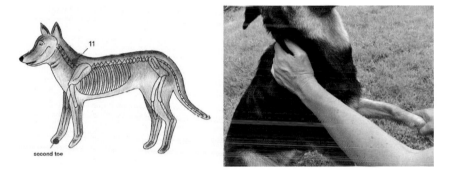

Or use the hold for initial centering (p. 19) by holding **SEL 10** together with **SEL 13**.

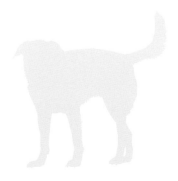

THROAT

Throat Infection (Laryngitis)

Place one hand on **SEL 11** and with the other hand hold the second toe of the front paw on the other side of the body (p. 159). Or place one hand on **SEL 11** and the other hand on **SEL 13** on the other side of the body.

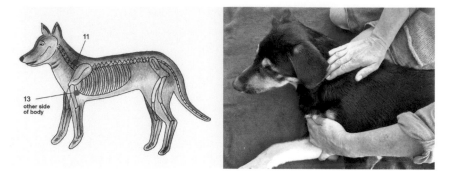

Laryngeal Catarrh

See "Throat Infection (Laryngitis)."

Or place one hand on **SEL 10** and the other hand on the crook of the elbow (**SEL 19**).

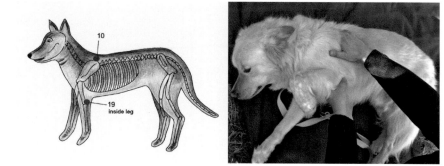

Cough and Chest Cold (Bronchitis)

Place one hand on **SEL 10** and the other hand on **SEL 19** (p. 160). Or hold **SEL 14** together with **SEL 22**.

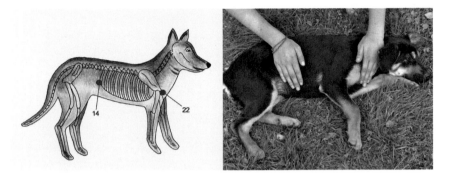

The initial centering hold (**SEL 10** and **SEL 13**) also helps relieve coughing and bronchitis.

Dry Cough

In order to specifically relieve dry cough, place your hands at a slight angle above **SEL 19** (inside of the front legs).

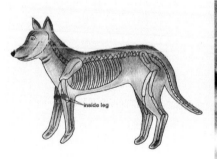
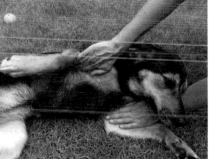

Lung Infection (Pneumonia)

To strengthen the lungs, hold **SEL 14** together with **SEL 22** (p. 161). Or hold **SEL 3** (the so-called antibiotic point) together with **SEL 15**.

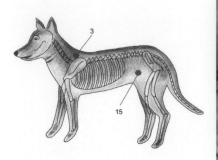

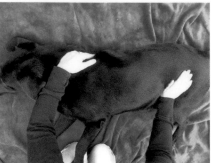

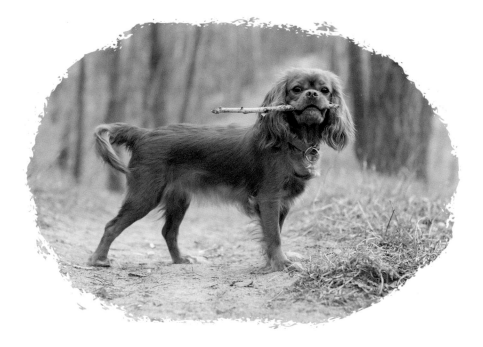

Digestive Organs

STOMACH

The stomach flow is suitable for all issues related to the stomach (p. 39).

Stomach Pain and Colic

To relieve colic, place your hands on both **SELs 1**, on the inside of the knee joints on the hind legs.

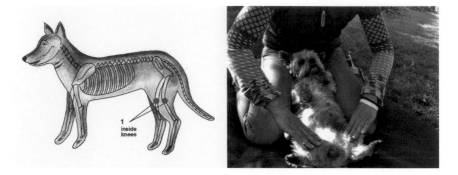

Or hold high **SEL 1** (approximately one paw's width above **SEL 1**) together with low **SEL 8** (approximately one paw's width below **SEL 8**).

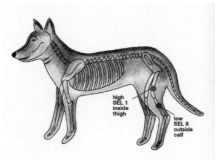
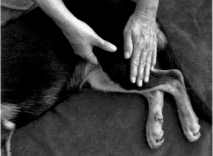

Vomiting

Hold both **SELs 1**. Or place one hand on **SEL 1**, the other hand on **SEL 14**.

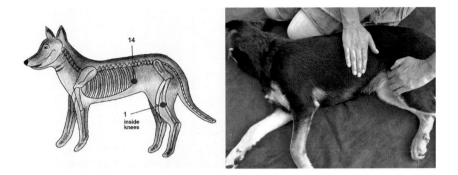

Twisted Stomach (Gastric Torsion)

Gastric torsion is more common in large dogs, especially Great Danes, shepherds, setters and St Bernards, although other dogs are not immune to it. Insufficiently tight connective tissue can slacken the suspension system of internal organs, in this case that of the stomach, which can then "rotate" due to factors such as increased gas formation. In such instances, only surgery will help.

You can also support your dog by holding both **SELs 15** or **SEL 15** together with **SEL 11** before and after surgery.

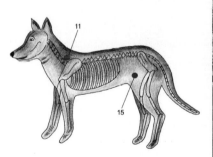
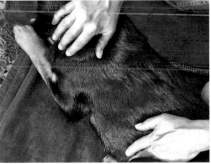

To prevent gastric torsion, or if gastric torsion has already been operated on, use the spleen flow (p. 35) regularly. The spleen flow keeps the organs in their respective places.

To strengthen the connective tissue, hold **SEL 16** together with **SEL 25** on a regular basis.

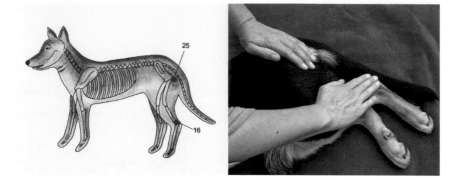

Loss of Appetite

The spleen flow (p. 35) harmonizes all eating behavior. It helps with loss of appetite, rejection of food, increased appetite, insatiable appetite, eating of rubbish etc. The stomach flow (p. 39) also helps to balance appetite and weight.

Weight Loss

The stomach flow (p. 39) and the spleen flow (p. 35) are also suitable here. Remember that the cause of weight loss can also be due to intestinal parasites (weight loss with normal appetite and eating behavior, p. 169) or thyroid diseases.

PANCREAS AND SPLEEN

To strengthen the pancreas, hold both **SELs 14**.

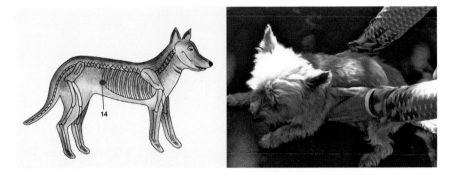

Or place one hand on **SEL 14** and the other hand on high **SEL 1** (about a paw's width above **SEL 1**) on the other side of the body.

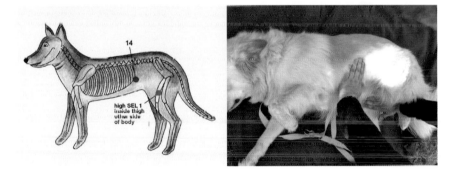

And to strengthen and support the spleen, use the spleen flow (p. 35). The spleen flow also supports the pancreas.

INTESTINE

Constipation

The cause of constipation is often a lack of exercise or an unvaried diet, unless serious illnesses are involved. Also, make sure that your dog always has access to fresh drinking water.

> To clear a blockage, hold both **SELs 1** (p. 217). Or place one hand on the second toe of the front paw and the other hand on **SEL 11** on the other side of the body.

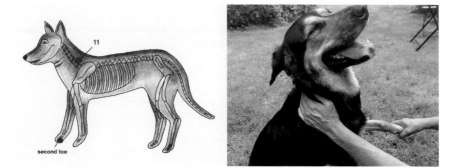

Diarrhea

Diarrhea can have a number of causes. If it does not improve within a day despite treatment, and/or the general condition of your dog is impaired, have it looked into by a vet.

> Hold both **SELs 8** or place one hand on the right **SEL 8** and the other hand on the right high **SEL 1** (about a paw's width above **SEL 1**).

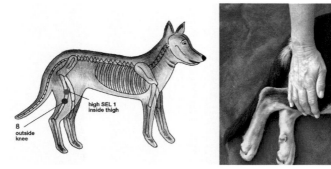

Intestinal Colic

To calm the bowels, you can place one hand on **SEL 1** and the other hand on high **SEL 19** on the other side of the body.

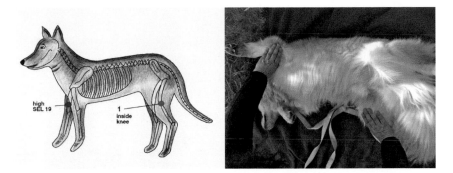

Intestinal Parasites

If your dog keeps having parasite issues, hold both **SELs 19** on a regular basis.

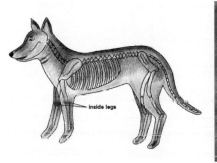
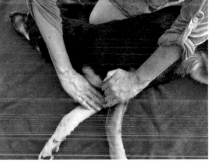

Or hold **SEL 3** together with **SEL 19** first on one side of the body, then on the other.

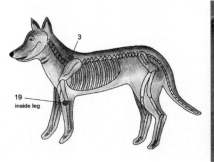
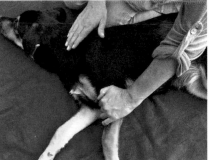

Blocked Anal Glands

Place one hand on the center of the neck on top of both **SELs 12** and the other hand on the tailbone.

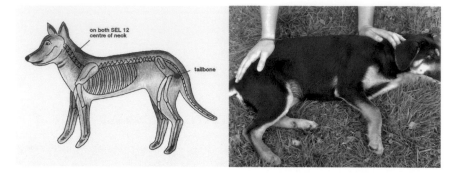

Hemorrhoids and Anal Fissures

Place one hand on the anal region and the other hand on **SEL 8**. Or hold **SEL 14** together with **SEL 15**.

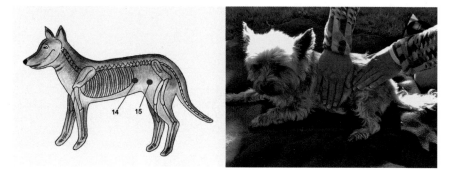

LIVER

To strengthen the liver, place one hand on the left **SEL 4** and the other hand on the left **SEL 22**.

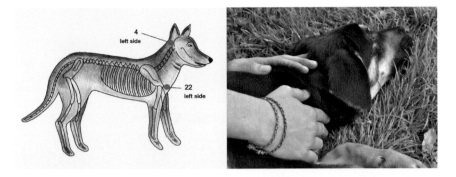

To detox, place one hand on **SEL 12** and the other hand on **SEL 14**.

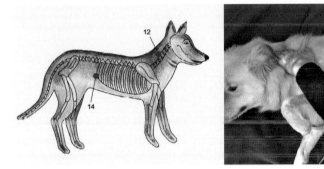

Or hold **SEL 23** together with **SEL 25**.

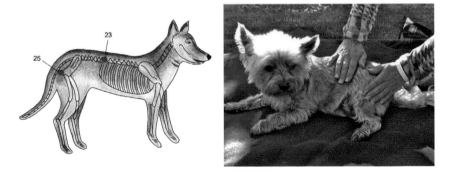

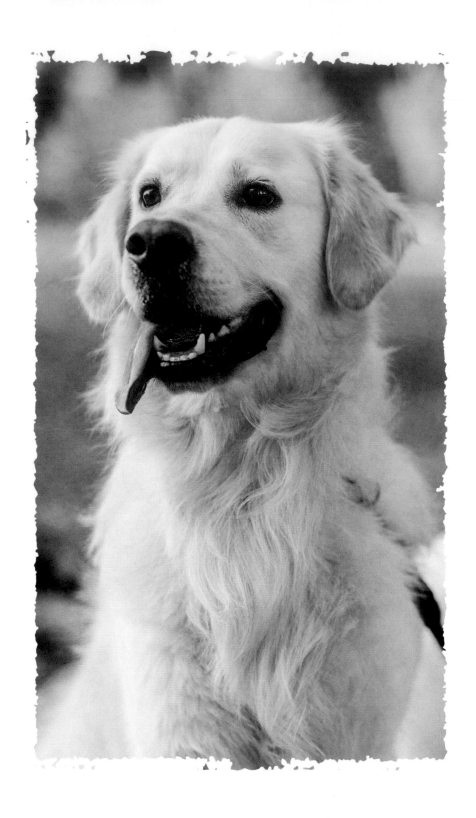

Musculoskeletal System

BACK AND SPINE

The so-called chiropractor flow involves the following holds:

Place one hand on **SEL 2** and the other hand on **SEL 6**. Do this on one side of the body and then on the other.

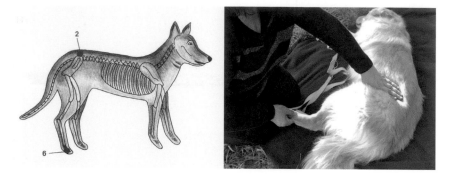

An important flow for all back issues is the bladder flow (p. 48). The paw flow (p. 22) also harmonizes the back and intervertebral discs.

MUSCLES

The following holds support the muscles and help with sore muscles, over-exertion, tremors, too high or too low muscle tone, strains, muscle pain, etc.:

Place one hand on **SEL 8** and with the other hand hold **SEL 5** together with **SEL 16**.

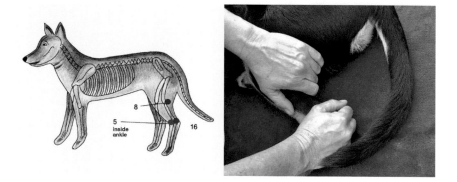

Or hold **SEL 8** and **SEL 5** first and then **SEL 8** and **SEL 16**.

To strengthen weak muscles, hold the left **SEL 12** together with the right **SEL 20**. And vice versa for the other side of the body.

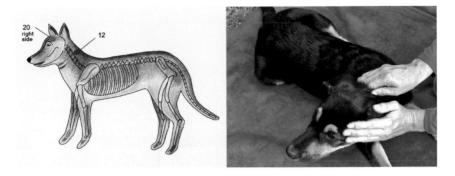

LIGAMENTS, TENDONS, AND JOINTS

Sprains and Strains

In cases of sprained hind paws hold the front legs at the first joint. With a sprained front paw hold the affected joint itself.

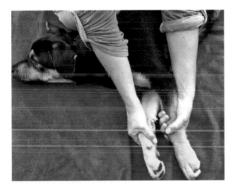

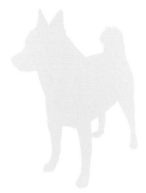

Or put one hand on the affected area and the other hand on **SEL 15** on the same side of the body.

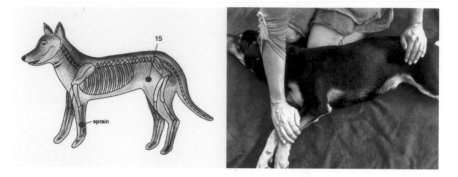

Strengthening Ligaments and Tendons

To strengthen ligaments and tendons, hold **SEL 12** together with **SEL 20** on the other side of the body (p. 178). Or place one hand on **SEL 4** and the other hand on **SEL 22** on the same side of the body.

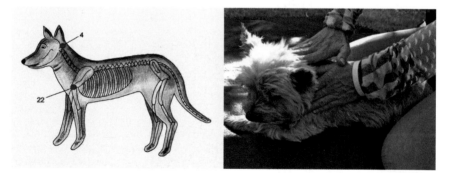

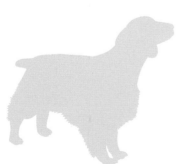

Joint Inflammation (Arthritis)

Use the detox hold regularly (p. 171).

To relieve the pain and heal the inflammation, hold **SEL 5** and **SEL 16** with one hand and **SEL 3** with the other hand.

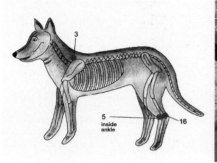
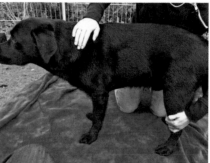

Joint Abrasion (Osteoarthritis)

Hold **SEL 13** and **SEL 17**.

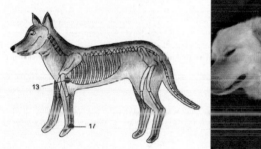
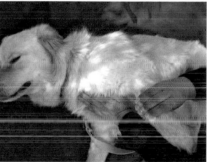

Treating **SEL 1** brings movement and agility. You can hold this point together with high **SEL 19** (about a paw's width above **SEL 19**) on the other side of the body.

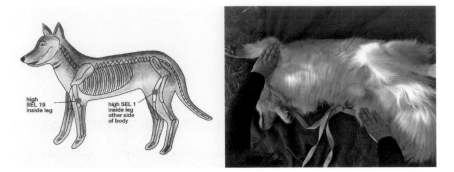

Hip Arthrosis

For the left hip, place your *left hand* on top of the left **SEL 12** and the *right hand* on the right **SEL 20** (p. 175). And vice versa for the right side of the body.

BONES

Broken Bones

Hold **SEL 15** to aid healing in broken bones; place both hands on the groin regions. You can also treat **SEL 15** together with **SEL 3**.

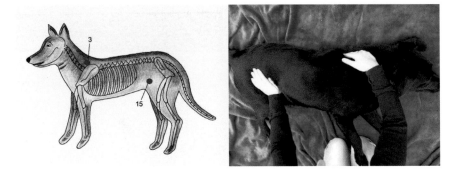

Strengthening Bones

To strengthen the bones, hold **SEL 11** together with **SEL 13** on the other side of the body.

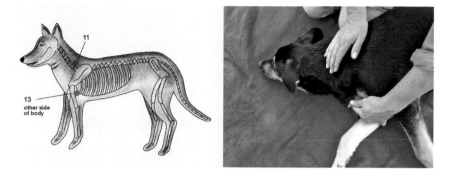

Or place one hand on the pubic bone and the other hand, in turn, on the two little toes of the hind feet.

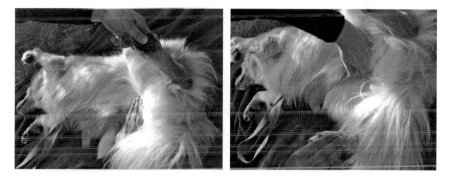

Growth Disorders and Bone Deformities

Hold both **SELs 18**.

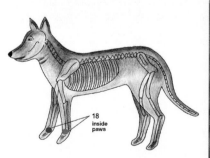
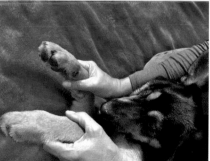

Or treat **SEL 25** together with **SEL 3**.

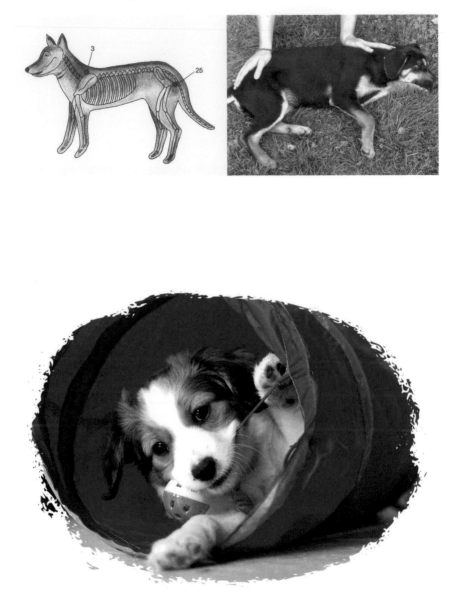

Urinary System

BLADDER

With all bladder issues (e.g., inflammation, paralysis), harmonize the bladder flow (p. 48). Or do the following quickies:

Place one hand between both **SELs 12**, in the middle of the cervical spine, and the other hand on the tailbone.

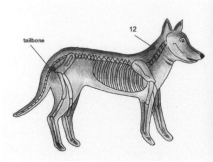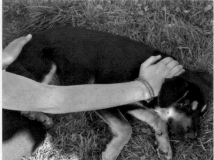

Or treat **SEL 4** together with **SEL 13**.

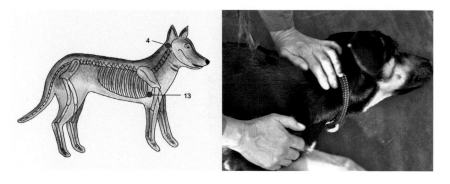

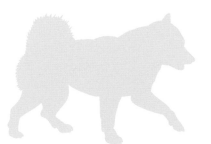

KIDNEYS

Kidney Infection

Hold **SEL 3** and **SEL 15** first.

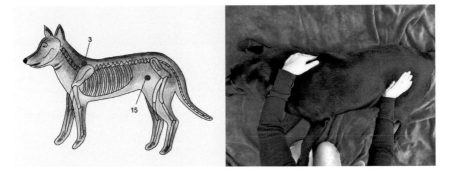

Then place one hand on the pubic bone, the other hand in turn on both of the little toes of the hind paw.

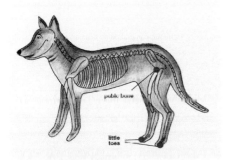

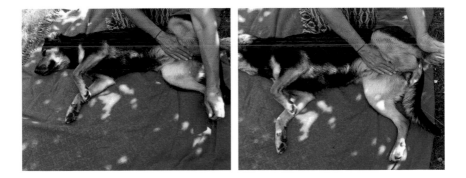

If your dog does not want to be touched on the pubic bone, place one hand on the back of the neck between both **SELs 4** and the other hand on the tailbone.

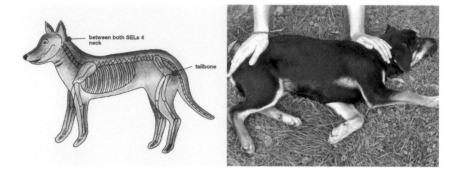

Kidney and Bladder Stones

Hold **SEL 5** and **SEL 16** with one hand and **SEL 23** with the other hand. Do the holds first on one side and then on the other side of the body.

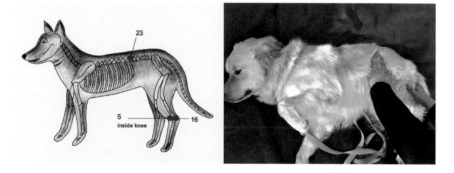

Or treat **SEL 23** together with **SEL 14**.

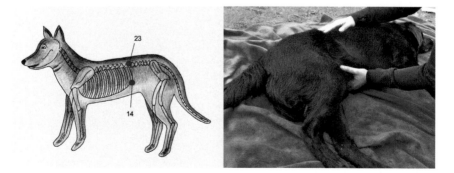

Reproductive Organs

Male Reproductive Organs

Female Reproductive Organs and Birth Support

MALE REPRODUCTIVE ORGANS

Inflammation of Testes (Testitis)

Hold **SEL 5** together with **SEL 16** with one hand and place your other hand on **SEL 3**.

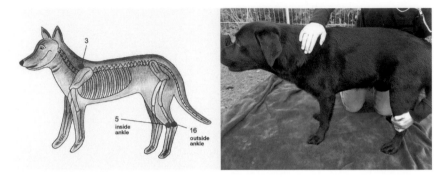

Prostate

Strengthen the spleen flow (p. 35). Place one hand between both **SELs 13**, on the sternum, and the other hand on the tailbone.

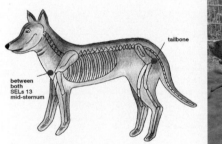
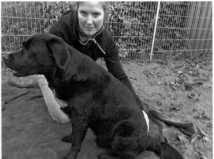

Excessive Sex Drive

Hold **SEL 19** together with **SEL 14** on the other side of the body.

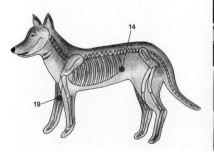
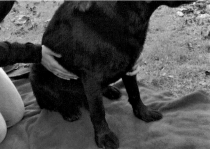

FEMALE REPRODUCTIVE ORGANS
AND BIRTH SUPPORT

Pregnancy

SELs 22 are important energy locks for adapting to a new situation (pregnancy, birth and the time afterwards).

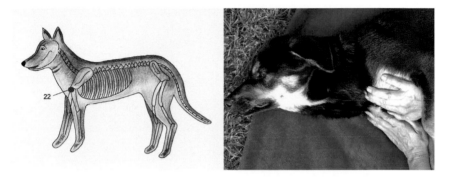

You can regularly use the supervisor flows (p. 31) during pregnancy.

SEL 5 held together with **SEL 16** supplies the uterus with energy.

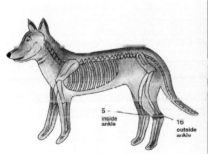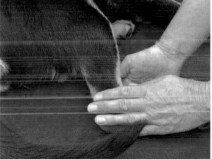

| 187

Prenatal Care

SEL 8 softens the pelvis for birth and opens the birth canal. **SEL 22** also prepares the body for birth. You can hold both energy locks together.

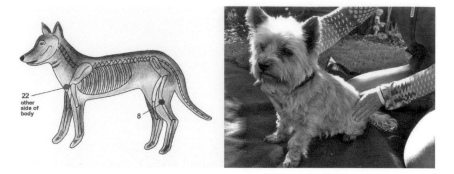

Birth Support

SEL 13 held together with **SEL 4** supports relaxation and a swift birth.

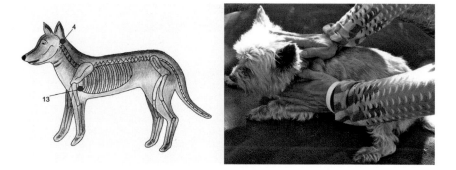

For general birth support and to promote contractions, place one hand on **SEL 8** (on either side of the body) and the other hand on the sacrum area.

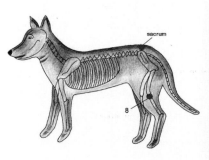
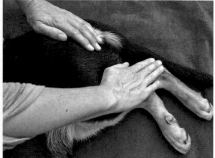

Labour Pains

Holding **SEL 5** together with **SEL 16** relieves pain during the birth (p. 187).

Too Weak or Too Strong Contractions

SEL 1 (p. 17) sets everything in motion and as such aids the entire birth process.

If the delivery stalls, or progresses too quickly, hold **SEL 20** and **SEL 21**.

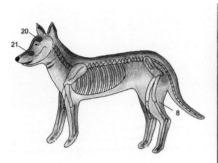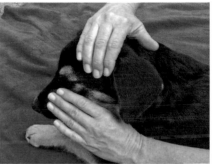

Breathing Issues in Newborn

If the newborn has breathing issues, hold both **SELs 4** (p. 17).

Milk Shortage or Surplus

To regulate the flow of milk, use the spleen flow (p. 35). Or place one hand on **SEL 22** and the other hand on **SEL 14**.

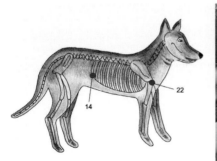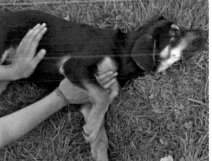

Inflammation of Teats

First, place one hand on **SEL 3** and the other hand on **SEL 15** (p. 183). Then hold high **SEL 19** (about one paw's width above **SEL 19**) together with high **SEL 1** (about one paw's width above **SEL 1**).

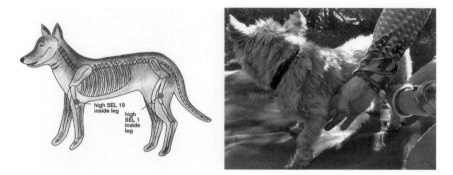

Pseudo-Pregnancy

Hold **SEL 10** together with **SEL 13** first on one side and then on the other side of the body. Or hold the area between both **SELs 10** with one hand and place the other hand on the chest in the area between both **SELs 13**.

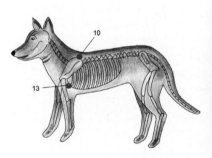
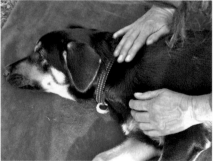

Sterility

Strengthen **SEL 13**: to do this, hold both **SELs 13** or **SEL 8** together with **SEL 13** on the other side of the body.

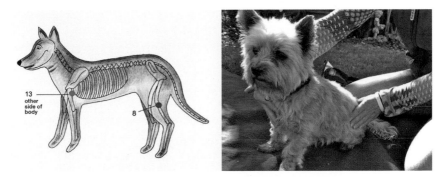

Strengthen the bladder flow (p. 48) and the spleen flow (p. 35).

Regulating Heat Cycles

Regularly use the spleen flow (p. 35) and the main central flow (p. 22).

Hold both **SELs 13**, or place one hand in the middle of the chest between both **SELs 13** and the other hand on the tailbone.

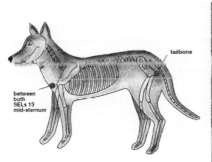
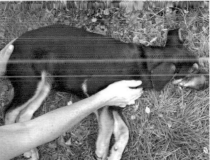

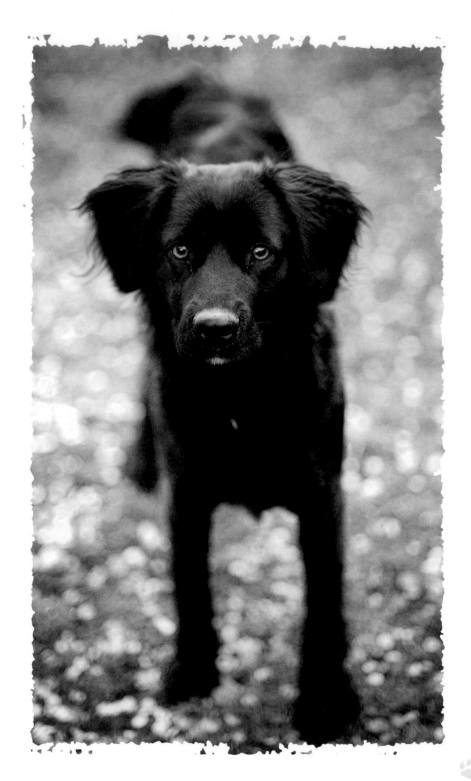

Coat and Skin

The stomach flow (p. 39) is the skin and hair specialist. If your dog has skin or coat issues, it is a good idea to use this flow regularly. Also, make sure your dog has a healthy and balanced diet.

COAT

Hair Loss

In addition to nutrition, a de-acidified body and an intact hormone system are important for healthy coat growth. Use the detox holds (p. 171).

To harmonize the endocrine system, treat **SEL 14** together with **SEL 22** on the other side of the body.

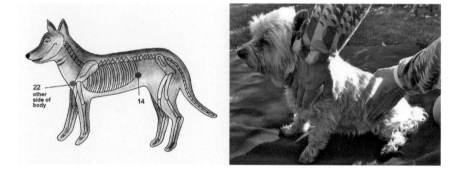

Dull Coat

In cases of a dull coat, regularly use the spleen flow (p. 35).

Dandruff

If your dog suffers from dandruff, harmonize the stomach flow (p. 39) and the spleen flow (p. 35).

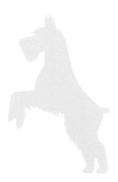

SKIN

Eczema

Regularly hold **SEL 3** together with **SEL 19**.

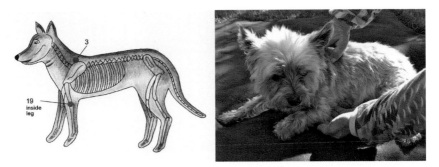

You can also hold **SEL 14** together with **SEL 22**.

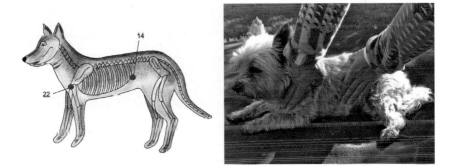

Boils and Abscesses

For boils and abscesses, and for everything that needs to get out of the body, place your *left hand* on the affected part of the body and your *right hand* on the *left hand*.

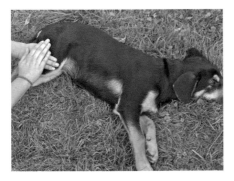

If you are in the company of others, you can also apply a "mountain of hands": place your *left hand* on the abscess and the *right hand* on the *left hand*, the next one places their *left hand* on your *right hand* and their *right hand* on the *left hand* etc. This speeds up the healing process.

Itching

To relieve itching, hold **SEL 3** together with **SEL 4**.

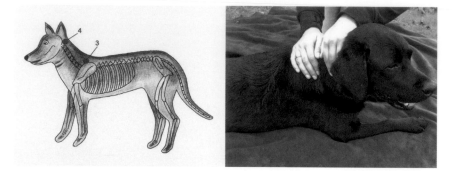

Allergies and Intolerances

Allergies are nowadays not only a common issue for humans, but also for dogs. There are different factors that can trigger an allergy, and often we can only guess at what the root cause may be. In allergies, the immune system is fighting substances that it should not be fighting.

With all allergies, the harmonization of the immune system is essential. **SEL 3** is the key to a well-functioning immune system. It is, so to speak, the door that swings open so that viruses and bacteria can leave the body again and through which the body can receive new, purified energy.

Hold **SEL 3** together with **SEL 15**.

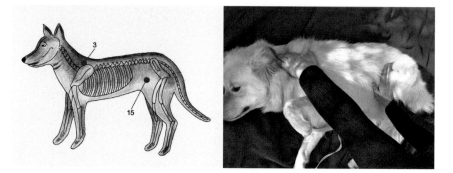

The spleen flow (p. 35) also strengthens the immune system. Another important hold for allergies is the following:

Place one hand on **SEL 19** and the other hand on **SEL 1**.

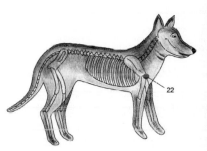
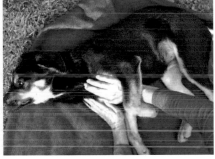

SEL 22 is an essential energy lock for all intolerances. It supports adaptation in a positive way. Hold both **SELs 22**.

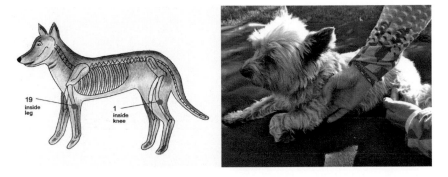

Or hold **SEL 22** together with **SEL 14**.

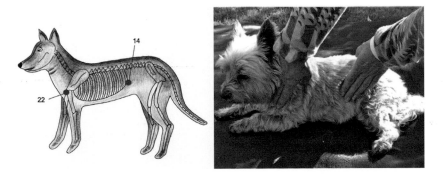

The initial centering hold is also very helpful (**SEL 10** and **SEL 13**, p. 20).

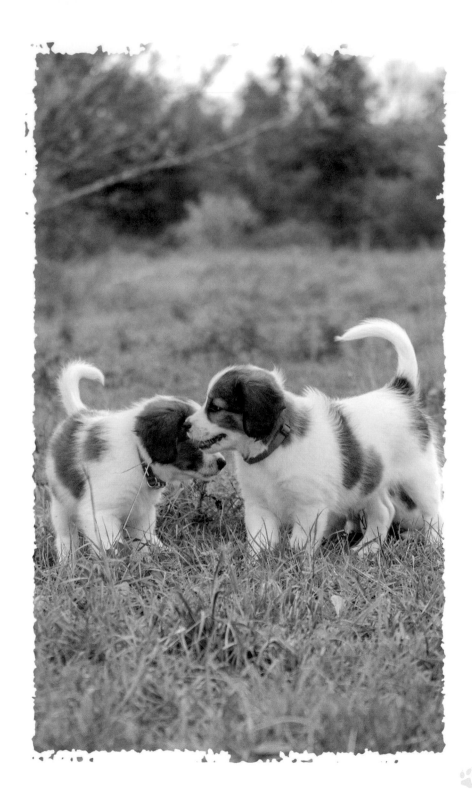

Nervous System

NEURALGIA

The stomach flow is suitable for neurological disorders in the head area (p. 39).

To relieve pain, hold **SEL 5** together with **SEL 16** (p. 187). Or hold **SEL 10** together with **SEL 17**.

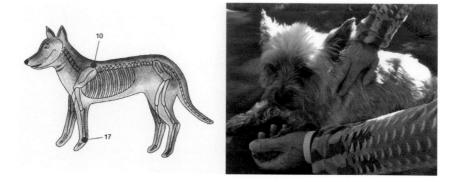

MUSCLE TWITCHING

Muscle twitching can be an accompanying symptom of various neurological diseases. This includes disorders in the nervous system as well as in the nerve cells of the muscles. Have this checked out by a vet.

It is not always caused by a disease. Muscle twitching is often harmless. Sometimes this symptom is also due to temporary nerve irritation.

Hold **SEL 8** together with **SEL 17**.

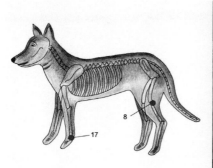
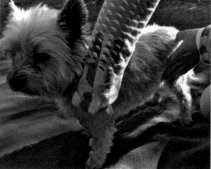

PARALYSIS

In cases of paralysis, use the following holds in turn:

For the right side of the body:
Place your *left hand* on the right **SEL 4** and your *right hand* on the right
  SEL 13.

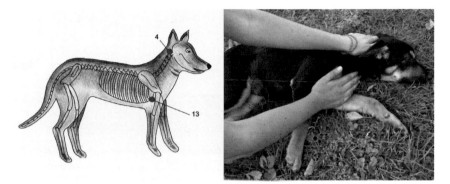

Then place your *left hand* on the right **SEL 16** and your *right hand* on the right
SEL 15.

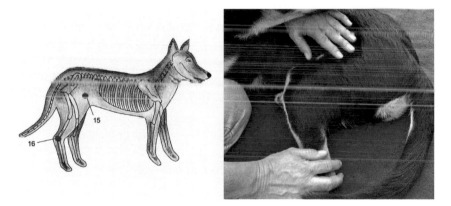

For the left side of the body, reverse the holds:
Place your *right hand* on the left **SEL 4** and your *left hand* on the left **SEL 13**.
Then place your *right hand* on the left **SEL 16** and your *left hand* on the left
SEL 15.

EPILEPSY

If your dog has epilepsy, you can support treatment in the following way:

Hold both **SELs 7** (the big toes of the hind paws).

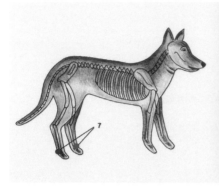 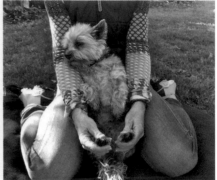

Hold neck and forehead frequently.

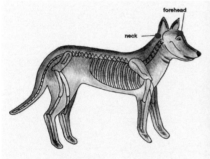 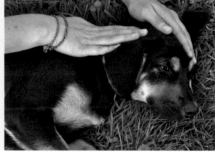

Hold **SEL 12** together with **SEL 14**.

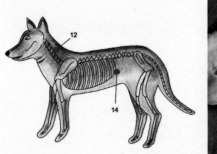 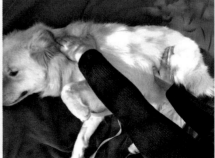

IMMUNE SYSTEM

An intact immune system is a prerequisite for health and vitality. As soon as you treat your dog, you automatically strengthen its immune system and stimulate its self-healing powers. The most important SEL for your dog's well-functioning immune system is **SEL 3**. When **SEL 3** is open and energy can flow through it unhindered, bacteria and viruses, which are in actual fact always present in the body, can leave the body again without getting stuck and triggering diseases.

You can also stop and dissolve incipient infections by opening **SEL 3**. The best way to do this is to hold **SEL 3** together with **SEL 15** (p. 196).

These flows further harmonize the immune system very effectively and powerfully:

- the main central flow (p. 22)
- the supervisor flows (p. 31)
- the spleen flow (p. 35)

Or hold **SEL 19** together with the high **SEL 19**.

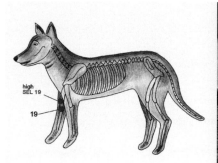
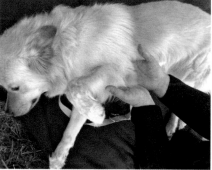

Infectious Diseases

If one of these potentially very serious diseases shows up despite vaccination, you can support your dog with flows in addition to veterinary treatment.

DISTEMPER

Susceptibility to distemper varies. It is said that mostly young dogs are affected, but older animals can also become infected. The first symptoms are often not recognized as distemper: a slight increase in temperature with tonsillitis, eyelid conjunctivitis and diarrhea with apathy. This phase can be quite harmless. Often the disease is only recognized in the second phase, which is usually more severe. This often leads to coughing, sneezing, nasal discharge, diarrhea and sore eyes.

Distemper can also disappear after the first two phases, if it takes a particularly mild course. However, all the aforementioned symptoms may fail to appear and instead the nervous system may be affected immediately. As a result, meningitis, an affliction of the spinal cord, failure of cranial nerves, epileptic seizures, rhythmic muscle tremors or cramps can occur.

In addition to veterinary treatment, give your dog a lot of support. It is best to use only very short flows for a few minutes, but more frequently throughout the day.

> Practise gentle flows like the supervisor flows (p. 31). Frequently hold **SEL 3** together with **SEL 15** (p. 196) and for detoxification hold **SEL 23** and **SEL 25** (p. 171). Strengthen the immune system (p. 204). And treat the points that are affected by the symptoms in question.

LEPTOSPIROSIS

Leptospirosis, also known as "Stuttgart disease," is an affliction that in acute cases quickly becomes fatal. It manifests through vomiting and diarrhea (usually including blood), rapid weight loss, foul-smelling breath, pain in the abdomen and high fever or low temperature. An antibiotic must be administered as quickly as possible.

> You can support the treatment by holding **SEL 3** and **SEL 15** several times a day (p. 196). Also hold both **SELs 1** (inside knee of hind legs) or **SEL 1** together with **SEL 8** (p. 168).

PARVOVIRUS

The parvovirus infection usually breaks out very suddenly and is associated with violent vomiting and accompanied or shortly followed by diarrhea, which is often bloody and watery. The greatest danger is dehydration and rapid weight loss.

In addition to veterinary treatment, treat the right **SEL 8** and left high **SEL 1** (p. 168). Apply the supervisor flows (p. 31) and hold the points to strengthen the immune system (p. 204).

KENNEL COUGH

Treat the points described in the section on cough and chest cold (p. 161). Apply the supervisor flows (p. 31) and generally strengthen the immune system (p. 204).

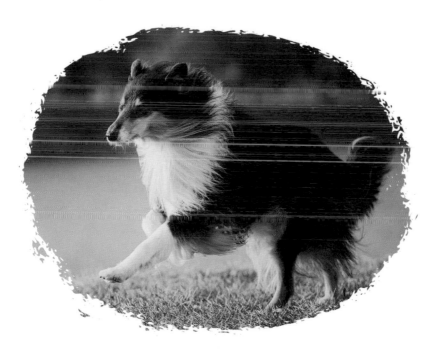

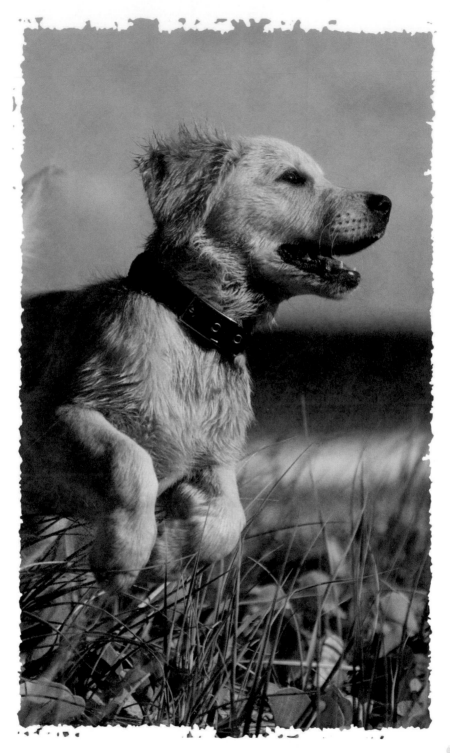

Edema, Growths, and Tumors

EDEMA

To dissolve edema, apply the bladder flow (p. 48).

GROWTHS AND TUMORS

Where there is movement, there can be no accumulation. Treatments bring energy flow back into motion, so that all that is old and hardened can be loosened. Jin Shin Jyutsu harmonizes the whole being and gradually brings everything back into balance – including cell growth.

> **SEL 1** (inside knee of hind legs), the original mover, sets everything into motion and dissolves blockages and accumulations.

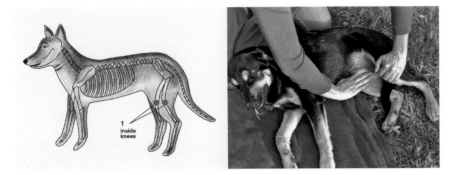

The spleen flow (p. 35) brings light into every cell and can dissolve tumors and accumulations. Apply the main central flow regularly (p. 22).

> Hold **SEL 20** on one side and **SEL 19** on the other side and then vice versa. This is an important hold for cell renewal.

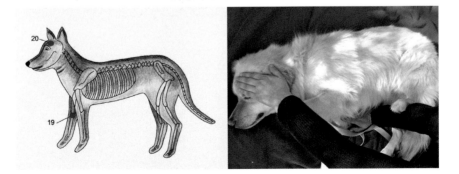

Use the supervisor flows regularly (p. 31). Detoxify the body (p. 171).

Hold **SEL 11** and the second toe of the hind paw on the other side of the body.

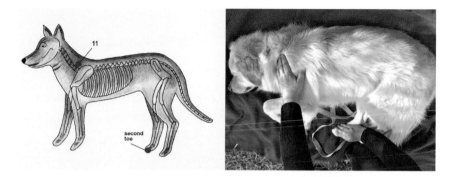

An important hold with malignant tumors and also effective for cysts is the following:

Place one hand on **SEL 24** (harmonizes chaos) and the other hand on **SEL 26**.

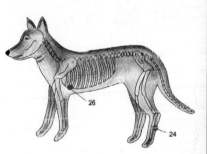
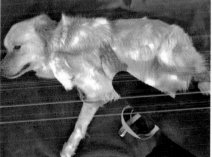

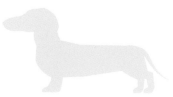

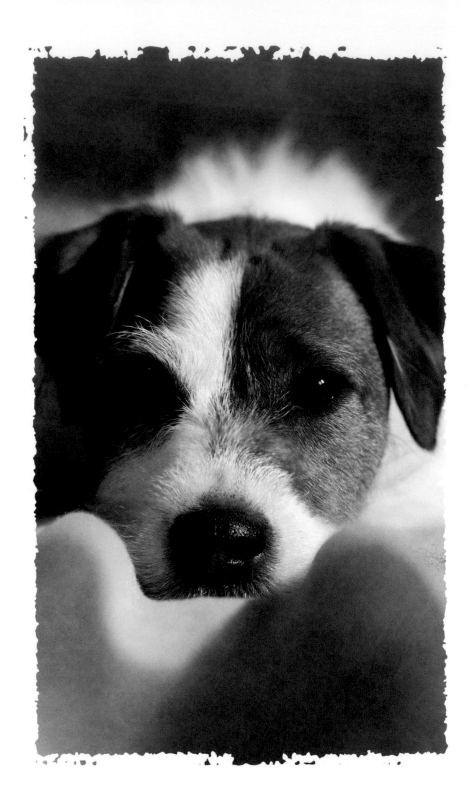

Injuries and Emergencies

Bleeding Wounds

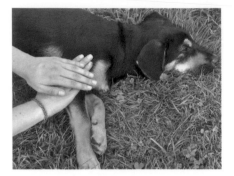

For bleeding wounds, place your *right hand* on or over the wound or dressing and your *left hand* on top of your *right hand*.

Festering Wounds

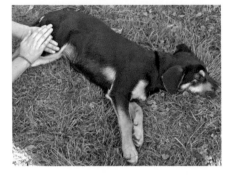

For festering wounds, place your *left hand* on or over the wound or bandage and your *right hand* on top of your *left hand*.

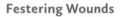

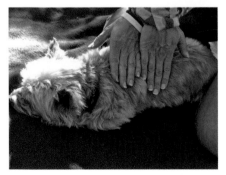

Cross your hands so that the little fingers are touching. Then place your crossed hands on the affected area.

BITES

See "Wounds" (p. 214).

STINGS, SPLINTERS, AND THORNS

Place your *left hand* on or over the affected area and your *right hand* on top of your *left hand*.

BURNS

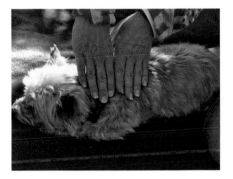

Place both hands side by side over the affected area.

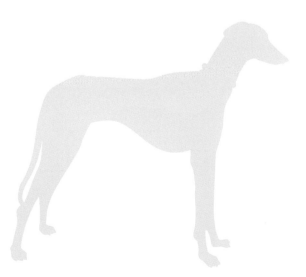

CONCUSSION

First hold both **SELs 4** and then both **SELs 7**.

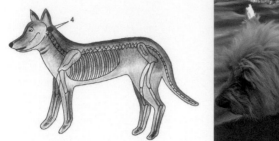

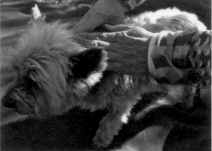

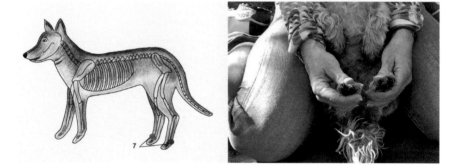

BROKEN BONES

Place both hands on the groin, on **SEL 15**, or place one hand on the broken bone and the other hand on **SEL 15**.

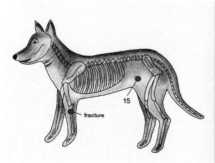

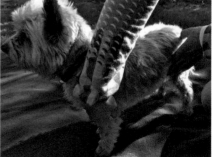

BRUISES

Place your *right hand* on the affected area and your *left hand* on top of the *right hand* (p. 214).

SHOCK

Shock is a life-threatening affliction of the circulatory system and without exception an affected animal belongs in the hands of a vet. Shock can be caused by a number of things, including heatstroke, injury, profuse bleeding, biting, poisoning, allergies, burns and twisting of the stomach.

Signs of shock are: your dog is weakened; rapid, shallow breathing; accelerated heartbeat; noticeably pale gums; paws, ears and tip of the tail feel cool; trembling; staggering.

For first aid, treat both **SELs 1** (inside knee of hind legs).

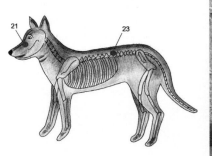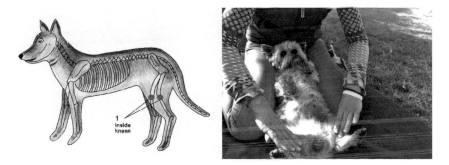

POISONING

In the event of poisoning, a vet must be consulted immediately.

Hold both **SELs 1** as first aid (see above). Also hold **SEL 21** and **SEL 23**.

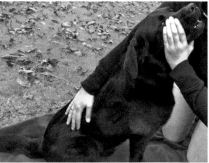

HEATSTROKE AND SUNSTROKE

The first aid holds for too much sun or heat are:

Hold both **SELs 4** (p. 216). Hold both **SELs 7** (p. 216).

CHOKING AND SHORTNESS OF BREATH

Hold both **SELs 1** (p. 217) or **SEL 1** together with **SEL 2**.

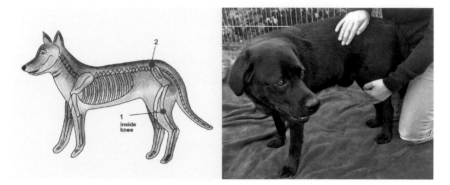

CRAMPS

Hold both **SELs 8**. Or hold **SEL 8** together with **SEL 1** on the other side of the body.

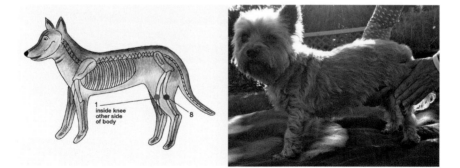

OPERATIONS

Hold both **SELs 15** before and after surgery.

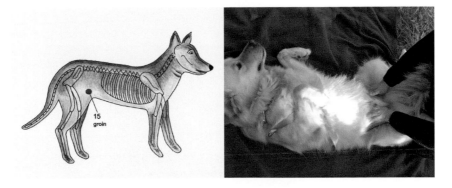

TRAVEL SICKNESS

Hold both **SELs 14** or hold **SEL 14** together with **SEL 1** (p. 165).

Pain

You can relieve all kinds of pain by holding **SEL 5** together with **SEL 16**, either first on one side of the body, then on the other, or by holding **SEL 5** together with **SEL 16** with each hand (p. 187) .

OVEREXERTION

Hold **SEL 15** together with **SEL 24**.

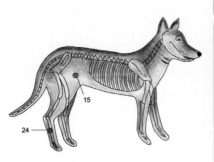
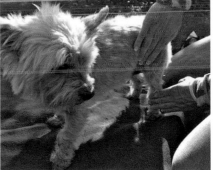

END-OF-LIFE CARE

To make the transition easier for your dog, hold **SEL 4** together with **SEL 13**. You can also treat both **SELs 4** with one hand and both **SELs 13** with the other hand.

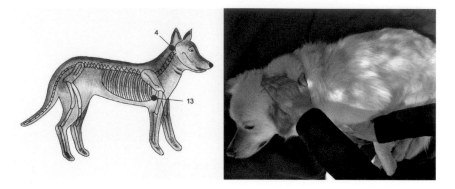

SEL 4 is an important energy lock that supports all transitions. It is said that it "stops the process of dying, if it is not yet time to die," and it helps those who are dying to pass over.

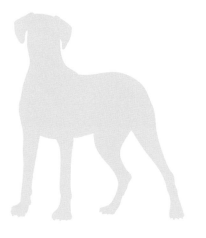

Psychological Issues

An important flow for treating fears is the main central flow (p. 22). It brings everything back to the center and evokes deep trust. **SELs 21, 22** and **23** are important energy locks for all issues related to fear. You can use these energy locks in the following combinations:

For the left side of the body:
Place your *right hand* on the left **SEL 21** and your *left hand* on the left **SEL 23**. If your dog does not like being treated in the face, hold **SEL 12** instead of **SEL 21**.

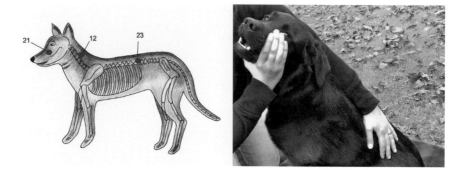

Then leave your *left hand* on the left **SEL 23** and place your *right hand* on the left **SEL 22**.

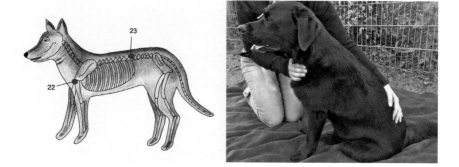

Reverse the sequence for the right side of the body:
First place the *left hand* on the right **SEL 21** or **SEL 12** and the *right hand* on the right **SEL 23**. The *right hand* remains on the right **SEL 23** and the *left hand* goes to the right **SEL 22**.

Another flow to harmonize fears is the following:

Place the *left hand* on the left **SEL 4** and the *right hand* on the left **SEL 12**. Then place the *left hand* on the left **SEL 12** and the *right hand* on the left **SEL 11**. For small or medium-sized dogs, you can hold **SEL 4** with one hand and **SEL 11** together with **SEL 12** with the other hand.

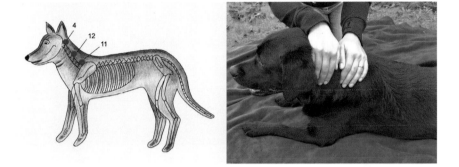

For the right side of the body:

First place the *right hand* on the right **SEL 4** and the *left hand* on the right **SEL 12**. Then place the *right hand* on the right **SEL 12** and the *left hand* on the right **SEL 11**.

INSECURITIES

For very insecure or nervous dogs, hold **SEL 17** together with **SEL 18** on one or both front legs simultaneously.

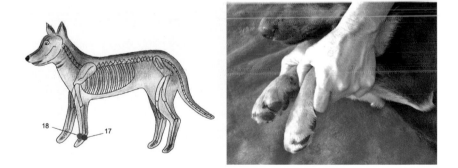

If your dog is very insecure and anxious, apply the main central flow (p. 22) regularly.

NERVOUSNESS AND STARTLE RESPONSES

Here, too, the main central flow (p. 22) is of great help. You can calm very nervous or frightened animals by holding both **SELs 1**(p. 217).
Or place one hand on **SEL 23** and the other hand on **SEL 26**.

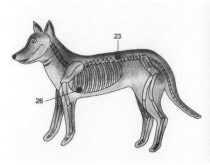
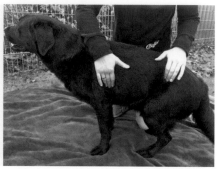

Or hold **SEL 21** and **SEL 22**.

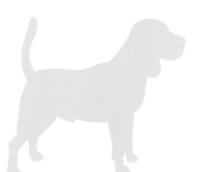
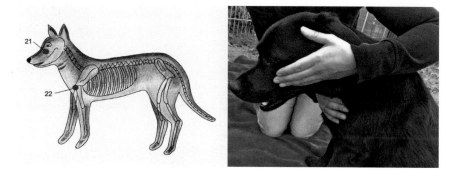

HOMESICKNESS

To relieve homesickness, hold both **SELs 9** (see drawing below on the left) or both **SELs 19** (see photo below on the right). This will help your dog adapt to new situations.

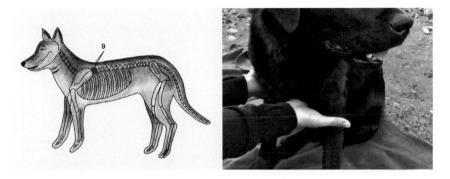

You can also hold **SEL 11** together with **SEL 12**.

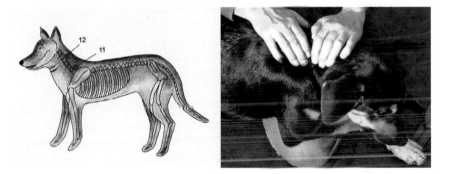

Or you can put one hand on **SEL 9** and the other hand on **SEL 11** and **SEL 12**.

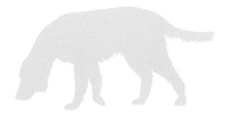

JEALOUSY

A helpful flow for jealousy is the stomach flow (p. 39).

Or hold **SEL 14** together with **SEL 24**. **SEL 24** harmonizes chaos – including internal chaos.

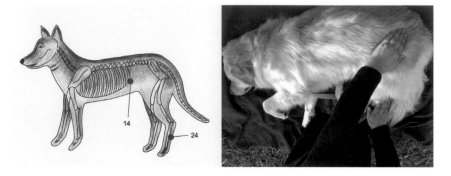

You can also hold **SEL 14** together with **SEL 22** (p. 197). **SEL 22** helps your dog adapt to given circumstances or situations.

FOOD ENVY

Hold **SEL 14** and high **SEL 19** (about a paw's width above **SEL 19**).

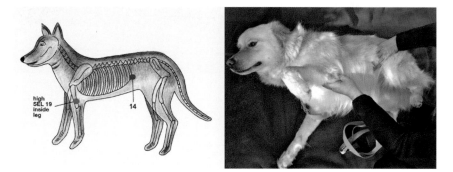

The stomach flow (p. 39) also brings relaxation and calm in this instance. Or, preferably, harmonize **SEL 13** together with **SEL 10** (see initial centering, p. 20).

FIGHTING AND AGGRESSION

If your dog is rather aggressive and gets quickly involved in fights, ensure good basic harmonization, e.g., by using the main central flow (p. 22).

Hold both **SEL 24**s or **SEL 24** together with **SEL 26**.

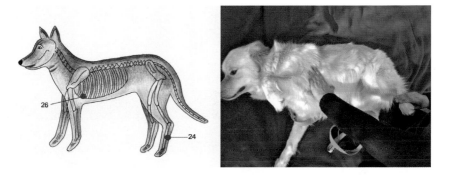

Hold **SEL 22** and **SEL 4** on the other side of the body.

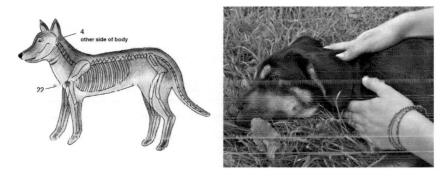

Hold **SEL 20** and **SEL 4** on the other side of the body.

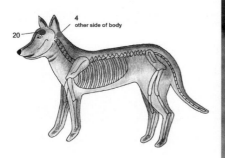
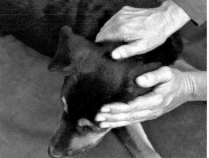

STUBBORNNESS

Hold **SEL 24** with **SEL 26** (p. 227) or with **SEL 12**.

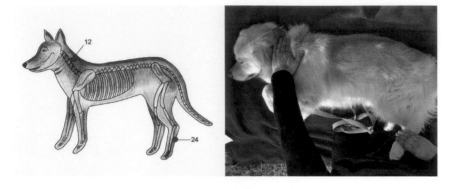

NEGLECT

If your dog has been neglected in its previous home, you can harmonize this imbalance with the spleen flow (p. 35).

ABUSE

Here, too, as with the issue of neglect, the spleen flow (p. 35) is an important flow for healing. The stomach flow (p. 39) relaxes, supports emotional healing and helps to rebuild trust. The hold for initial centering (p. 20), holding **SEL 10** together with **SEL 13**, also helps the dog to process negative experiences one step at a time.

Hold **SEL 22** and **SEL 4** on the other side of the body.

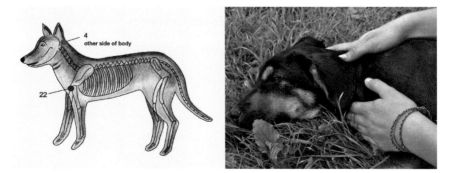

Hold **SEL 20** and **SEL 4** on the other side of the body.

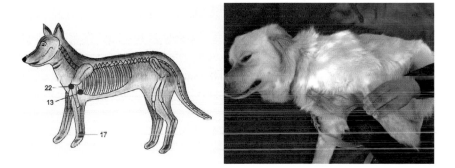

SENSITIVITY TO NOISE

If your dog is very sensitive to noise, you can support it by placing one hand on **SEL 22** and **SEL 13** at the same time and holding **SEL 17** with the other hand – first on one side of the body and then on the other.

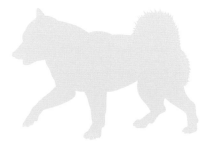

The spleen flow (p. 35) also helps with hypersensitivity of all kinds.

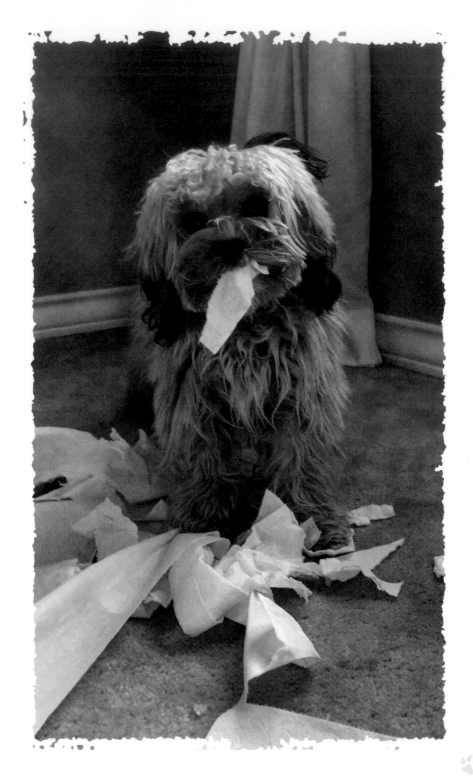

Other Issues

HOUSE-TRAINING

The bladder flow (p. 48) helps your dog to better control and regulate its excretions.

EATING RUBBISH OR FECES

There are different opinions as to why many dogs eat feces. Some assume that pet food attractants or flavourings in pet food make feces so attractive for dogs, whereas others interpret it as a sign of mineral deficiency. However this may be, it is an unpleasant thought for humans and unhealthy for a dog to eat feces, as it can ingest parasites and become infected with diseases. The more balanced and harmonious a dog is, the more it will eat what is good for it. Still, there are always exceptions, as dogs have their own mind – or idea of what is delicious. For a balanced appetite, strengthen the stomach flow (p. 39). Likewise the spleen flow (p. 35) harmonizes eating behavior.

LACK OF CLEANLINESS

If your dog is a bit careless with its grooming, you can support it by holding **SEL 12** (one hand between both **SELs 12** in the middle of the neck) and the tailbone (at the base of the tail).

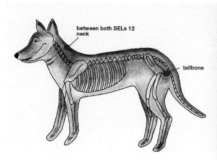
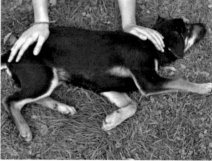

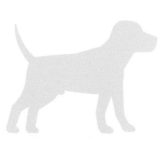

HARMONIZING SIDE EFFECTS OF MEDICATION

To compensate for the side effects of drugs, hold **SEL 21** and **SEL 23** first on one side and then on the other.

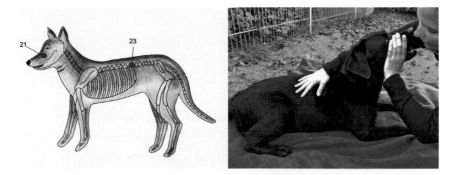

Hold both **SELs 22** or **SEL 22** together with **SEL 23**.

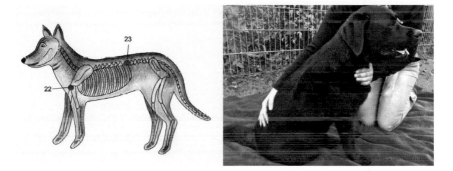

ALLEVIATING REACTIONS TO VACCINES

Use the spleen flow (p. 35) so that the immune system is strengthened and can thus deal better with harmful substances.
Or hold **SEL 23** and **SEL 25**.

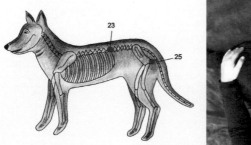
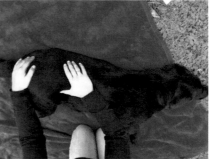

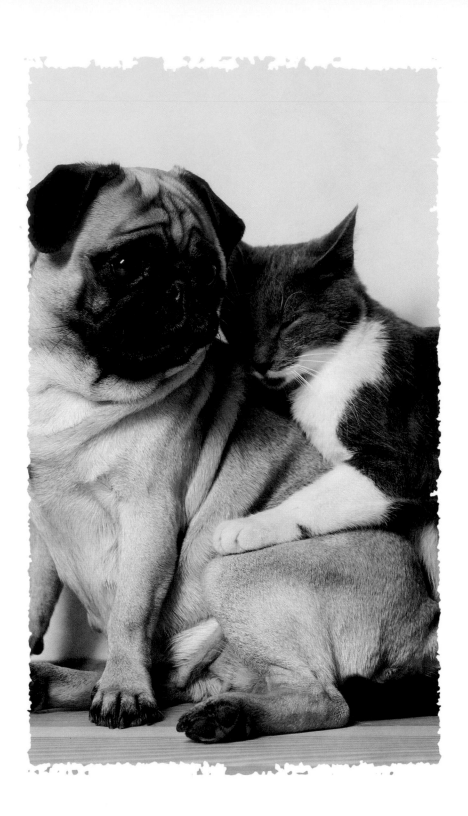

Epilogue

S tay tuned! Jin Shin Jyutsu, the art of the creator for compassionate people, is a wonderful, simple and yet highly effective method to strengthen yourself and your pet in all situations. It is best to make a habit of treating your pet as well as yourself daily – even if only briefly. As you harmonize imbalances, life energy regains momentum, self-healing powers are activated and symptoms can resolve themselves once more. Your pet visibly feels better. It is more relaxed – and of course healthier!

You can use Jin Shin Healing Touch to prevent illnesses and to support the healing process for existing illnesses, injuries, etc. It also strengthens your relationship with your pet – and with yourself. What is more, it does not need to take up a lot of time, since animals react very quickly to being treated. Usually a few minutes are enough. You yourself will also feel strengthened and more relaxed afterwards.

Wishing you further wonderful experiences with Jin Shin Jyutsu! Heartfully,

Tina Stümpfig

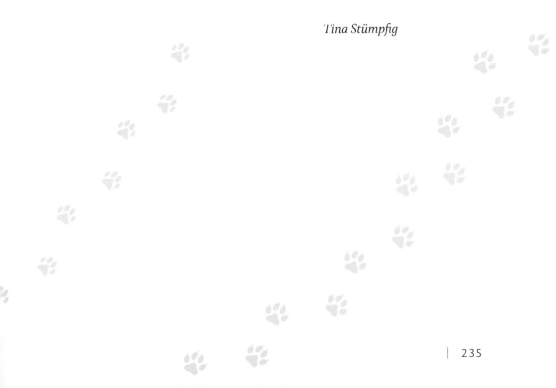

Acknowledgements

I thank Jiro Murai, who rediscovered Jin Shin Jyutsu and passed on his knowledge of this art, and Mary Burmeister, who brought this knowledge to the Western world, disseminating it with love and thereby making it accessible to us all. I would like to thank all the teachers with whom I was, and am repeatedly, allowed to study.

A big thank you goes to my father, Erwin Weber, for the cat and dog drawings. I would like to thank all the photo models – people, dogs and cats – for their support: Ronja and Nola with Carlos, Annette with Isabella and Kitty, Tanja with Darwin, Sonja with Knut, and my daughters Jana, Mira, Samaya and Lucia with Mirkosch, Luna and Shila.

Thank you to everyone who embarks on the "Jin Shin healing touch adventure" with their animals for your love and patience. Thank you to all who apply, share, and pass on Jin Shin Jyutsu without reservation, reminding themselves and others over and again that the greatest treasure lies latent within us.

Photo Credits

Jin Shin photos Cats & Dogs © *Tina Stümpfig*
Jin Shin illustrations Cats & Dogs © *Erwin Weber*

Decorative photos, interior:
P. 5: unlimphotos # 9157210 (© cynoclub);
P. 7: unlimphotos # 1047034 (© cynoclub);
P. 8: dreamstime # 22536535 (© Lilun);
P. 10: shutterstock # 1992708143 (© Natalia Bachkova);
P. 12: dreamstime # 139525962 (© Andreykuzmin);
P. 18: shutterstock # 211771213 (© Jagodka);
P. 30: shutterstock # 1043814685 (© Tatiana Gladskikh);
P. 34: elements-envato # 39WYL4N (© Elegant01);
P. 56: elements-envato # KHFUQ84 (© photocreo);
P. 67: elements-envato # PG6SN5X (© Corina Daniela Obertas);
P. 68: elements-envato # DNRDAPA (© twenty20photos);
P. 74: elements-envato # PCPGQ2F (© lightpoet);
P. 78: elements-envato # PK5AATN (© oxygen2608);
P. 92: shutterstock # 1568473846 (© newsony);
P. 100: elements-envato # 67V38N4 (© Sonyachny);
P. 106: elements-envato # SQUX52M (© gstockstudio);
P. 110: elements-envato # KT3V4DF (© Sonyachny);
P. 118: elements-envato # RGVZDA9 (© twenty20photos);
P. 122: elements-envato # Z5LSAL9 (© ivankmit);
P. 126: dreamstime # 95817189 (© Dachux21);
P. 140: elements-envato # KDHYECK (© twenty20photos);
P. 142: unlimphotos # 40296006 (© tan4ikk1);
P. 156: elements-envato # PHUVHDD (© EpicStockMedia);
P. 162: elements-envato # VTAFX6J (© fotyma);
P. 172: elements-envato # 4TLL8VS (© bernardbodo);
P. 180: elements-envato # SPVY75E (© twenty20photos);
P. 192: elements-envato # PA4EDLL (© halfpoint);
P. 198: elements-envato # 2G77KY3 (© twenty20photos);
P. 207: elements-envato # EERZP9C (© Grigory Bruev);
P. 208: elements-envato # PQL38HL (© mvaligursky);
P. 212: elements-envato # WAE3FK9 (© twenty20photos);
P. 230: elements-envato # DYHZNWJ (© twenty20photos);
P. 234: shutterstock # 538300048 (© Studio Africa).

Cover images: elements-envato # P9AYREA (© CreativeNature_nl);
www.depositphotos.com # 83785848 (© Konstanttin); # 104019110 (© aksenovko);
www.shutterstock.com # 388713619 (© adtapon duangnim).

Recommended Reading

Burmeister, Alice. *The Touch of Healing: Energizing the Body, Mind, and Spirit with Jin Shin Jyutsu*. New York: Bantam Books, 1997.

Burmeister, Mary. *Introducing Jin Shin Jyutsu Is, Books 1–3*. Scottsdale, AZ: Jin Shin Jyutsu, Inc., 1980.

———. *What Mary Says: The Wisdom of Mary Burmeister*. Audio edition. Scottsdale, AZ: Jin Shin Jyutsu, Inc., 1997.

Fahrnow, Ilse-Maria. *Mehr Energie mit Jin Shin Jyutsu*. Munich, Germany: Südwest Verlag, 2012.

Leas, Adele. *Jin Shin Jyutsu for Your Animal Companions*. New Orleans, LA: Self-published, 2004.

Riegger-Krause, Waltraud. *Health Is in Your Hands: Jin Shin Jyutsu – Practicing the Art of Self-Healing*. New York: Upper West Side Philosophers, Inc., 2014.

———. *Jin Shin Jyutsu – Einfache Anwendung zur Selbsthilfe*. Munich, Germany: Südwest Verlag, 2005.

Stümpfig, Tina. *Jin Shin Healing Touch: Quick Help for Common Ailments*. Rochester, VT: Findhorn Press, 2020.

Stümpfig-Rüdisser, Tina. *Meine Hände helfen und heilen*. Petersberg, Germany: Verlag Via Nova, 2008.

———. *Lebensquell Jin Shin Jyutsu*. Petersberg, Germany: Verlag Via Nova, 2010.

———. *Jin Shin Jyutsu – Die Kunst des Heilströmens erlernen*. Petersberg, Germany: Verlag Via Nova, 2013.

———. *Jin Shin Jyutsu – Heilbehandlung bei Tieren*. Petersberg, Germany: Verlag Via Nova, 2015.

About the Author

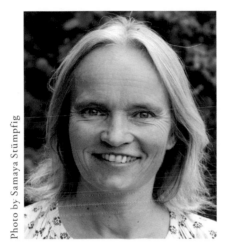

Photo by Samaya Stümpfig

TINA STÜMPFIG, psychologist and special education specialist, has been working as a Jin Shin Jyutsu practitioner with humans and animals for many years. In individual treatments as well as in group seminars, she shows that everything we need to be happy and healthy lies within ourselves. The author of *Jin Shin Healing Touch: Quick Help for Common Ailments*, Tina has written several textbooks on the subject of Jin Shin Jyutsu.

For more information visit: **www.tinastuempfig.de**